What Do These Women and Children Have in Com

T0106946

- A 3-year-old boy exhibits severe dev ceives a diagnosis of autism…

- A 28-year-old woman is unable to conceive …

- A 6-month-old baby develops therapy-resistant seizures…

- An 8-year-old boy is prescribed Prozac because of odd, uncontrollable behavior…

- A 12-year-old boy slowly loses his ability to walk and write, becoming bedridden…

- A 9-month-old baby stops responding to his parents and can no longer sit up by himself…

- A 38-year-old mother is condemned to life in a wheelchair after gastric bypass surgery…

- A 7-year-old boy has obsessive-compulsive behaviors, and a wide-based gait…

- An 18-year-old can't concentrate or understand her instructors and drops out of her first semester of college…

- A 9-year-old girl needs to attend a special school for handicapped children because she has an IQ of 60…

- A 15-year-old teen becomes severely depressed and tries to kill herself…

- A 31-year-old with severe postpartum depression has thoughts of harming her infant…

Here's what these patients *don't* have in common: a correct diagnosis. Instead these women and children have been given a plethora of incorrect, often hopeless diagnoses: developmental delay, autism, depression, multiple sclerosis, Asperger's syndrome, cerebral palsy, attention deficit disorder, and mental illness. But in reality, they all suffer from the same medical condition…

Vitamin B₁₂ Deficiency

COULD IT BE B12?
PEDIATRIC EDITION

What Every Parent Needs to Know
About Vitamin B$_{12}$ Deficiency

Sally M. Pacholok, R.N., B.S.N.
Jeffrey J. Stuart, D.O.

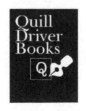

Fresno, California

Could It Be B$_{12}$? Pediatric Edition
Copyright © 2016 by Sally M. Pacholok and Jeffrey J. Stuart.
All rights reserved.
A previous edition of this book was published as
What's Wrong with My Child? (ISBN 978-1-61035-244-4)

Published by Quill Driver Books,
an imprint of Linden Publishing
2006 South Mary, Fresno, California 93721
559-233-6633 / 800-345-4447
QuillDriverBooks.com

Quill Driver Books and Colophon are trademarks of
Linden Publishing, Inc.
ISBN 978-1-61035-287-1
first printing
Printed in the United States of America
on acid-free paper.

Library of Congress Cataloging-in-Publication Data on file.

Acknowledgments

We would like to thank the many dedicated physicians, researchers, and other clinicians who have contributed a vast amount of medical documentation regarding the devastating effects of vitamin B_{12} deficiency in children and adults.

We are grateful to the Groovers, the Ryans, and other families who recognized the importance of sharing their stories about their children's B_{12}-deficiency-acquired injuries in order to educate others. Special thanks go to Tracey and Damian Witty in the United Kingdom, who teamed up with **www.B12Awareness.org** to educate more countries about the dangers of B_{12} deficiency—there is power in numbers.

We are truly blessed to have the opportunity to work with writer, producer, and film director Elissa Leonard, who shares our passion and joined our lifelong quest to raise public awareness and expose poor health-care practices through her movie *Sally Pacholok*.

A big thank you to Chris Kelley, president of Polestar Communications, who taught me the fundamentals of giving a great interview and writing pitches. His continued support, advice, and friendship are priceless. Thanks also to Ron Beckenfeld, Matthew Supkoff, Steve Downs, Greg Faull, and the rest of the team at Superior Source Vitamins for their past and continuing efforts on behalf of B_{12} awareness and educating the public. And finally a private thanks to my dear friends Tracy Weick, Karen O'Donnell, and Dr. Richard Nimbach—life would not be the same without your kinship, laughter, and listening ears.

Team B$_{12}$

The Groover Family
The Ryan Family
The Leone Family
Ron Beckenfeld
Jaguar Bennett
Alison Blake
David Carr, M.D.
Joseph Chandy, M.D.
Michelle J. Cheatley
Pauline Ciaffone
Jeffrey Dach, M.D.
John Dommisse, M.D.
Anna Dutko
Joseph Flynn, D.O.
Kelly and Jack
  Genzlinger
Susie Griffiths
Teddy Harasymiw
Suzie Henson-
  Amphlett
Martyn Hooper
Chris Kelly

Pat and Kim Kornic
Elissa Leonard
Priscilla Leone
Charles H. Liu, R.Ph.
Joshua Luckasavitch
Lulu Ann Mattocks
Kilmer McCully, M.D.
Glenn Medina
Hugo Miney, Ph.D.
Daria Mytyakynska
Richard Nimbach, D.O.
Eric Norman, Ph.D.
Karen and Mike
  O'Donnell
David R. Pacholok
Anna Pijanowska
Patrick Prentice
Kathy Reichenbach,
  R.N.
George and Donna
  Rossetti
Larry and Justyna
  Slabosz

Rick Solecki
Kent Sorsky
Anand Sridhar, Ph.D.
Heather Stratton,
  D.D.S.
Sue and John Stuart
Matthew Supkoff
Paul Thomas, M.D.
Alice and Carl
  Vandemergle
Carmen Velazquez,
  M.D.
Margaret Venske
Patricia Waldo
Tracy and Edward
  Weick
Tracey and Damian
  Witty
Linda and Ken
  Woolcock

In Memory of B$_{12}$ Angels

Dale and Charlene
  Back
Paul and Priscilla
  (Mickey) Bowman
Joannes Dutko, D.D.S.
Paul Fernhoff, M.D.
W. Michael Forgette,
  D.D.S.
Melinda Groover
Sue Harvey
John Hotchkiss, M.D.

Grace Izzi
Helen M. Kosy
Connie Lamb, R.N.
Matteo Leone
Brian Liska, D.O.
Milton and Jean Lute
Jim Mundy
Mary and Michael
  Nykiforuk
Andrew and Anna
  Pacholok

William and Nancy
  Pacholok
Samuel Radzik
Bernard Rimland,
  Ph.D.
Marie Rusconi
Mary and James Stuart
Edward Waldo
Daria Zakharko

Dedication

This book is dedicated to the memory of my beloved parents, Anna June and Andrew William Pacholok—you are always with me and on my shoulder. My parents were loving, encouraging, wise, and self-sacrificing. Their early teachings and example have allowed me to flourish, endure, and protect others.

This book is also in memory of wife, mother, and grandmother, Melinda Groover, who fought to bring awareness of B_{12}-related disorders to the public and prevent needless injuries. Melinda inspired us to create this special pediatric edition. Her love, friendship, spirit, advocacy, and Alabama charm, are all sweet reminders of a life well lived. She will remain forever in our hearts.

This book is also dedicated to all those who suffer from developmental, learning, and other neuropsychiatric disabilities as a result of B_{12} deficiency. Despite never conceiving a child or having been a "mother" in the truest sense, I have been given an equally important assignment in life by God: to prevent B_{12} deficiency, especially in vulnerable children and the elderly, and to help those already struggling with the consequences of late diagnosis. In my heart, all B_{12}-deficiency-stricken children and seniors are my children.

This book is dedicated as well to the memory of Dr. Bernard Rimland, whose support and encouragement were invaluable and whose passion lives through us. And it is dedicated to the memory of Sue Harvey and Grace Izzi, who spread the word about B_{12} deficiency in their hair salon from 2005 to 2013, educating and saving many women and their families. I know you are continuing to walk with me on this journey.

—Sally Pacholok

"Do not withhold good from those who deserve it, when it is in your power to act."

—**Proverbs 3:27**

"All truth passes through three stages. First, it is ridiculed. Second, it is violently opposed. Third, it is accepted as being self-evident."

—**Arthur Schopenhauer**

Contents

Foreword by George A. Rossetti

Vitamin B_{12} deficiency, and the myriad consequences and complications associated with it, ruins lives. I learned, the hard way, just how destructive an unrecognized, untreated B_{12} deficiency can be—from grim personal experience. It derailed my life, destroyed my career, and left me for disabled at 50 years of age. Were it not for the guidance, support, and kindness of authors Sally Pacholok and Jeffrey Stuart, I wouldn't be receiving the treatment I so desperately need, and you wouldn't be reading this foreword.

My humble contribution aside, what truly matters is that you are reading this book, because the information contained in these pages could prove life saving. I'm not given to exaggeration; it is important that this book be widely read . . . by parents, by the general public, and especially by physicians and others in the health-care community who are poised—whether they know it yet or not—to prevent suffering on a grand scale among their most helpless, vulnerable patients.

Seven months ago I had never even heard of Sally and Jeff, I knew nothing of their work, and they certainly had no idea who I was. That changed suddenly and dramatically on February 4, 2014. Four months prior, in October 2013, after I had suffered for over a decade from a host of baffling, increasingly debilitating neurological signs and symptoms consistent with multiple sclerosis, an astute neurologist I'd only recently met finally diagnosed me with advanced subacute combined degeneration (SCD) of the spinal cord and nervous system, one of many debilitating diseases caused by severe B_{12} deficiency. I finally knew the name of the fiend that put an end to my 30-year career as a medical writer in 2010, and continues to erode my ability to enjoy life or even accomplish simple tasks of day-to-day living.

Receiving an accurate diagnosis was challenging enough; getting proper treatment would prove nearly impossible. Vitamin B$_{12}$ deficiency, my neurologist informed me, is generally treated in the primary-care setting. She described a typical replacement regimen and said she would be happy to speak with my internist if he had any questions. Speed was of the essence; days and weeks matter once SCD is diagnosed. Unfortunately, many weeks would be lost before treatment could be started. Within days of receiving the verdict, I met with my internist, informed him of the diagnosis, and provided copies of supporting laboratory results and radiology reports. When I described a standard treatment protocol widely used to correct the deficiency, his jaw dropped. "That's an awful lot of B$_{12}$," he gasped, then summarily refused to have any hand in treating me and declined to discuss the matter further. "You're on your own with that," he announced. And so I was. Another physician I subsequently approached likewise balked.

Owing to my years in medical publishing, I had considerable resources at my disposal and knew how to use them. I scoured the medical literature, identified a commonly used replacement regimen, acquired a sizeable quantity of cyanocobalamin and the means to deliver the injections, and then went to work. After three months of following the treatment protocol faithfully, I felt even worse than I did in October. The numbness and tingling in my legs was advancing and now involved my hands and arms, an ominous sign of progression. I was weaker than ever, having problems walking and staying on my feet, and tremors were worsening. Forgetfulness, memory loss, and cognitive decline (so fatal to my career) remained serious problems. A sense of hopelessness settled in, I felt utterly defeated—then I met Sally Pacholok.

By chance, I saw Sally and Jeff in a documentary titled *Diagnosing and Treating Vitamin B$_{12}$ Deficiency*. The next day, consumed with frustration, I reached out to them via e-mail at their website (**B12Awareness.org**). My message was little more than a whining rant. I sought neither advice nor guidance. I simply described my symptoms (far more numerous than mentioned above) and told my sorry tale of medical mismanagement. I was venting, and never really expected a reply. I certainly wasn't expecting the reply I got.

Sally came right back at me, as an avenging angel riding the whirlwind of a gathering storm. (This rather florid metaphor will make excellent sense to those who know Sally.) Her compassionate, voluminous response contained a laundry list of questions—questions about my medical history, current treatment, medications past and present—you name it. I answered all to the best of my ability, feeling afterward as though I had just undergone a thorough, virtual physical examination. By day's end, Sally had me switched from cyanocobalamin to hydroxocobalamin. She gave me sound, credible reasons to believe that improvement was still possible, and for the first time since seeking treatment, I no longer felt I was "on my own." Barely 24 hours after establishing contact, I had become one of B_{12} Sally's Kids.

But I'm no kid, and this book isn't about me or my problems. This work exists solely to speak out for those who can't speak for themselves—our children, who can't necessarily describe or understand symptoms of B_{12} deficiency, who aren't equipped to take matters into their own hands when medicine abandons or neglects them, and who are at the mercy of a health-care community that far too often fails them. Because of my personal experience with this dread disease, the ignorance and arrogance I encountered in the medical community, and my extensive experience as a medical writer, Sally kindly invited me to read the manuscripts for this book and to contribute a foreword.

I felt at once honored and a bit anxious. One can't help but feel flattered when entrusted by an author to contribute so conspicuously to their work. I answered in the affirmative, without hesitation, and with great enthusiasm. I felt obliged to remind Sally, though, that consequences of a severe B_{12} deficiency forced me out of medical publishing years ago, and I haven't been at the top of my game for some time. But she was unconcerned, and soon I started receiving manuscripts bearing the text contained herein. My enthusiasm soon turned to despair, which grew more abject with every page I read.

Regardless of my history, current condition, or whatever struggles might lie ahead, I enjoyed 45 years of excellent health before lack of B$_{12}$ caught up with me. Compared with the youngsters portrayed in this book—true stories all—I'm a very lucky man. Yet it hardly cheers the soul to admit that. Sally and Jeff leave nothing to the imagination about how a combination of arrogance, negligence, and unforgivable ignorance—my words, not theirs—in the medical community is needlessly shattering fragile young lives, so often before they leave the cradle, and too often preventing them from ever doing so.

As an adult with SCD, possessed of a deep knowledge of medicine and human physiology, I understand the forces at work in my body. The mystery underlying the abnormal sensations, cognitive problems, and mood swings has at last been revealed. That knowledge alone is helpful. Life was far more difficult, indeed frightening, before I was correctly diagnosed. I know what I'm fighting now. But I simply can't fathom how horrifying the nightmare must be for uncomprehending children and desperate parents.

My wife Donna and I have no children; odds are high my B$_{12}$ deficiency is responsible for that particular deficit as well. Regardless, try as I might I can't imagine the pain and frustration parents must experience watching helplessly as a child withers before their eyes, while the physicians they trust stumble and stagger from one blind alley to the next, outpaced by the relentless hands of a clock. Time and Death wait for no physician.

Yet within these pages, you'll find examples of gifted, caring physicians who practice good medicine, who ask the right questions, and seek answers in likely places. Time and again, savvy physicians make the right call, pulling patients from the edge of the abyss, often just short of too late, and usually after another physician dropped the ball. You'll also read of far too many physicians who for any number of reasons—arrogance, pride, ignorance, incompetence—should never have been allowed near a stethoscope in the first place.

Medicine is art, not science. Its practitioners, like all artists, rely on science and technology to provide them with the tools and knowledge they need to practice their craft. Some artists are great; some, not so great. A mediocre sculptor might produce a bad monument, but nobody gets hurt. A bad physician is a menace to society. As the reports in this book clearly demonstrate, it pays to find the best providers available and be prepared to move on if red flags start to fly. If you suspect that you or a loved one might not be receiving adequate care, there's a good chance you're right.

Could It Be B₁₂? Pediatric Edition is concise, easy to read and understand, and contains a wealth of information no parent, grand-parent, aunt, uncle, or family friend should be without. It should certainly be required reading for all physicians. The truth—terribly simple and simply terrible—is that B_{12} deficiency cripples and kills. It is a color-blind assailant that claims and destroys the lives of men, women, and children, from all walks of life, and with equal enthusi-asm. This book is much more than a treatise on the consequences of B_{12} deficiency in children. It is a clarion call for simple change with far-reaching implications. It challenges all physicians to be more circumspect in making diagnoses, to recognize and abandon bad habits, and it argues emphatically and persuasively that tragedy can be avoided and lives saved by keeping one simple question in mind. Could it be B_{12}?

George A. Rossetti
Executive Editor (*Emeritus*), *Gastrointestinal Cancer Research*
Former Associate Editorial Director, *ONCOLOGY*

Foreword by Dr. Paul Thomas

Once or twice a year, a book comes along with a message so powerful, important, and life-changing that it becomes a "must read." *Could It Be B$_{12}$? Pediatric Edition* is just such a book.

If you or a loved one suffers from less than optimal health, you need this book. If you desire a long and healthy life, free from anxiety, depression, neurological problems, and vascular disease, you need to read this book. If your child has developmental delays, seizures, or any neurological or psychological issues, this book may just have the answers you have been looking for.

Clearly, vitamin B$_{12}$ is not the cure for all ailments. However, B$_{12}$ deficiency is an under-appreciated and widespread disease that contributes to many of the major health problems both children and adults are battling today. For example, this book clearly defines the connection between B$_{12}$ deficiency and the current epidemic of autism. While rising autism rates cannot and should not be blamed entirely on B$_{12}$ deficiency, there is no question in my mind that B$_{12}$ deficiency is far more prevalent than realized and can be a significant cause of or contributor to autism spectrum disorders.

My own youngest biological son was borderline autistic and had no focus in preschool and the early grades, resulting in severe learning and academic issues. After hearing a talk on B$_{12}$ deficiency by autism specialist James Neubrander, M.D., in 2002, I started my son on methyl-B$_{12}$ shots. Within a couple of months, he had gained two grade levels and was clearly no longer borderline autistic.

My own work in the area of autism and ADHD (I have about 1,000 patients with these diagnoses) has led me to believe that a major key to treating individuals with these disorders lies in minimizing toxins and maximizing nutrition. In this regard, B$_{12}$ is particularly crucial, because a lack of this nutrient causes damage to every system in the body—particularly the brain and nervous system. Moreover, B$_{12}$ plays a powerful role in defending against toxins. For example, individuals with *MTHFR* gene defects—which are very common, and reduce the body's ability to use vitamin B$_{12}$ and an associated vitamin, folic acid—have increased difficulty removing toxins from their bodies. As the toxins in our air, food, and water increase, these individuals are becoming far more vulnerable to developing autism and related disorders.

I confess that I was guilty of not having my son's B$_{12}$ levels tested prior to starting his treatment. I strongly agree with the authors that testing is important, not only to establish a diagnosis so treatment can be tailored to an individual patient, but also to help us understand the real prevalence of vitamin B$_{12}$ deficiency in children with autism and other neurological and psychiatric disorders.

The section on testing in this book is thorough and informative. Physicians, please read this and remember your training in basic science. Too often, physicians focus on treating a label such as autism or depression, when finding the real underlying cause can lead to a cure and prevent lifelong suffering.

This book makes a compelling case for the need to provide B$_{12}$ screening for all pregnant women, all infants, and anyone experiencing neurological or psychological symptoms. Testing is simple and inexpensive, and—as Sally and Jeff show—it not only can save lives but also can save billions of dollars for health-care systems around the world.

This book is a call to action for us all: physicians, legislators, parents, attorneys, and all patients who suffer from the physical and psychological symptoms caused by B$_{12}$ deficiency. It is a must read for every person who cares about health and wellness, and perhaps the most important health book I have ever read.

Thank you, Sally and Jeff, for shining the light on this major health crisis. I am hopeful we can all work together to end it.

Paul Thomas, M.D., FAAP, ABIHM, ABAM
Board certified in Pediatrics
Author of *Feel 20!*

Introduction

In 1985, I was formally diagnosed with juvenile autoimmune pernicious anemia, one of many causes of B_{12} deficiency. I had to fight to get a correct diagnosis, with two doctors dismissing my abnormal blood test results as "insignificant" and another doctor, a seasoned hematologist, writing in my medical record that I was "anxious" or slightly hysterical for thinking I had a problem. The hematologist arrogantly commented: "This is an old person's disease." I stood my ground, was inquisitive, and debated the doctor. My feistiness paid off in the end, because I eventually received an accurate diagnosis and correct treatment, saving me from disability or even death.

However, millions of people aren't as fortunate as I was. After I received my own diagnosis, I began doing extensive research into B_{12} deficiency—and what I found horrified me. Worldwide, I learned, this devastating disorder goes largely undiagnosed. As a result, people of all ages suffer terribly or even lose their lives. And those who do get diagnosed often don't get proper treatment.

I gained a personal perspective on this tragedy after I began working as a registered nurse in an emergency department in 1987. Again and again, I encountered patients who were symptomatic or at risk for B_{12} deficiency but did not receive testing. My anger and frustration rose as my efforts to educate doctors and administrators hit a brick wall. I knew my own health had once hung in the balance when I had to fight with my own doctors to get a correct diagnosis. Now, my patients needed someone to actively advocate for them. And so my B_{12} journey began.

As a nurse, I was appalled by the scale of the B$_{12}$-deficiency epidemic, and by the cost in human suffering and health-care dollars. But what I didn't realize at the time was that *even I was underestimating the scope of the problem*. And then a personal experience opened my eyes even further.

In the spring of 2000, the 3-year-old son of a member of my extended family received a diagnosis of autism. When I heard the news, I began scouring the Internet and libraries for information on this disorder. And as I researched autism, pulling up journal articles and reading medical texts, I discovered something startling: The signs and symptoms of autism in children were eerily similar to the signs and symptoms of B$_{12}$ deficiency.

At first, I simply thought I had tunnel vision because of my personal and professional interest in B$_{12}$ deficiency. But the more I read, the clearer the picture became. Doing literature searches, I uncovered case after case in which B$_{12}$ deficiency in infants and young children led to developmental delay or developmental regression. Published articles as far back as the early 1960s described autism-like signs and symptoms in children with B$_{12}$ deficiency, including speech and language delays, loss of skills, withdrawal, poor eye contact, self-stimulating behaviors, low IQ, and even seizures. Researchers who followed some of these B$_{12}$-deficient children after treatment found that they generally improved physically but remained cognitively delayed. When formally tested, these children were classified as "mentally retarded." Their treatment came too late, because their brains were injured due to a lack of B$_{12}$ during critical growth and development.

Could this be? Could infants and young children also be victims of a medical disorder that wreaks such havoc in adults? And could many developmentally delayed children with a diagnosis of autism actually have brain injuries caused by B$_{12}$ deficiency? Here is what I theorized in our first book, *Could It Be B$_{12}$?*, back in 2005:

It is interesting to note that signs and symptoms of B$_{12}$ deficiency generally seen in adults can also be seen in autistic patients. For example, undiagnosed B$_{12}$ deficiency in a 78-year-old can result in *behavior that includes dementia, babbling, psychosis, rocking, poor attention, and the appearance of "being in a separate world." The infant or toddler with undiagnosed B_{12} deficiency can also exhibit dementia, babble, have a poor attention span, appear unresponsive to the outside world, rock, or appear psychotic. The key difference between these two groups lies in their age and, thus, their stage of brain development. The adult has already acquired language, is wired for speech, and has a mature brain. The infant or toddler, in contrast, has not acquired or mastered speech or language, or passed through all the normal developmental stages. Therefore, the infant's or child's vocabulary and behavioral repertoire are more primitive, and symptoms will be expressed in a different way.*

In short, senior citizens with dementia could just as accurately be labeled as "autistic," and we could just as accurately label children with autism as "demented" or "senile." In all cases of adult dementia, B_{12} deficiency must be ruled out. However, we do not do this with autistic children because the medical community has not yet made the connection between the behaviors labeled as dementia and the behaviors labeled as autism.

In the years since we published our first book, we have uncovered a wealth of evidence clearly pointing to B_{12} deficiency as one significant cause of autistic behavior. It is now undeniable that many cases of autism are not autism at all, but instead what we refer to in this book as BABI: *B_{12}-deficiency Acquired Brain Injury*.

At a time when the incidence of autism is skyrocketing, it is shocking that doctors are unaware of the autism-B_{12} connection, and that virtually no children with autistic symptoms get tested for B_{12} deficiency. This is malpractice of the worst kind. Unlike autism, B_{12} deficiency is easy to diagnose and both simple and inexpensive to treat. Moreover, quick treatment can prevent permanent brain damage and reverse symptoms. Clearly, B_{12} deficiency isn't the explanation for every case of autism, but it *is* the explanation for many children—and those children deserve to be diagnosed.

However, as you will see, autism is far from being the only tragedy that can befall B$_{12}$-deficient children. In these pages, you will read stories about children and teenagers who suffered crippling symptoms, including blindness, crushing fatigue, learning disabilities, depression, psychosis, and suicidal urges, all because they were B$_{12}$-deficient. You will read stories about children who lost their ability to crawl or to walk. You will read stories about children who were diagnosed too late, and became permanently injured. And tragically, you will read about children who died.

B$_{12}$ deficiency doesn't just threaten your child's well-being or life; it threatens you and other members of your family as well. For example, we describe in this book parents who developed mental illnesses or became too physically ill to care for their children because they were low in B$_{12}$. We share information on how B$_{12}$ deficiency can cause postpartum depression or postpartum psychosis. And we show how a B$_{12}$ deficiency can make women infertile or cause them to miscarry. If you are pregnant, breastfeeding, or planning to become pregnant, this is information you need to know.

Of greatest importance, this book will give you the tools and information you need to protect your child's health. You'll learn how early diagnosis and treatment—efforts vigilant parents can take charge of—can lead to full or partial recovery. And you'll learn to identify the warning signs of B$_{12}$ deficiency, and how, if necessary, to get your child the tests and treatment he or she deserves.

This book was born out of necessity, passion, and a desire for justice. I was spared from the ravages of vitamin B$_{12}$ deficiency, and it is my mission to spare others as well—especially the precious, vulnerable infants and children who need us to be their advocates. I believe that as you read about this silent epidemic and its victims, you will become as infuriated as Jeff and I are over the massive failure of medical professionals and the government to protect the people whose lives are in their hands. And I hope that you will join us in spreading this crucial message: B$_{12}$ deficiency is common, it is dangerous, and *it is entirely preventable*. There is power in numbers, and if we band together, we can stop this dreadful epidemic in its tracks.

1

Vitamin B$_{12}$ Deficiency: A Silent Crippler Stalks Mothers and Children

As a mother or mother-to-be, you want to do everything possible to protect your child's health. In fact, it's your highest priority in life.

So imagine how devastated you'd be to learn your precious child was crippled for life. Then imagine learning that the disease that ruined your child's life is easy to diagnose and simple to treat—but doctors didn't bother to check for it. Or imagine discovering that you were suffering a significant deficiency when pregnant or nursing, and that both you and your child are at risk of developing devastating, lifelong consequences as a result.

For many parents, nightmares like these are a reality. These parents and their children face grim futures, because the doctors and hospitals they trusted missed one of the simplest diagnoses in medicine: vitamin B$_{12}$ (cobalamin) deficiency.

This crippling disorder can attack the human brain, nerves, blood cells, vascular system, and immune system at any age. In infants and children, it can cause developmental delay, behavioral problems, learning and intellectual disabilities, seizures, and brain injury. In people of any age, it can cause blood clots, leading to strokes, pulmonary embolisms, and deep vein thromboses. In pregnant women, it can cause miscarriages, preeclampsia, neural tube defects, and stillbirths. It can be an underlying cause of infertility in women encountering problems conceiving. In young children, it's often misdiagnosed as autism. And at any age, it can cause severe or even deadly anemia.

Many doctors mistakenly believe that B$_{12}$ deficiency is an "old person's disease," but it isn't. B$_{12}$ deficiency can strike any person at any age. It can destroy the health of a young adult, cause irreversible damage to a fetus during pregnancy, or cripple an infant, young child, or teenager for life. It can even kill.

This is especially tragic because B$_{12}$ deficiency is simple to identify, easy and inexpensive to treat, and can be simple to cure (though *not* with a standard vitamin pill or prenatal supplement, as we'll explain shortly). But it can be cured only if it is diagnosed and treated early. Unfortunately, that's the exception rather than the rule.

WHO ARE THE VICTIMS OF B$_{12}$ DEFICIENCY?

B$_{12}$ deficiency can strike people of any age, race, or economic class. Here's a sampling of cases from the medical literature:

- A 4-month-old baby develops therapy-resistant seizures.
- An 8-month-old baby loses her speech, stops responding to her parents, and eventually can't even sit up by herself.
- A 10-month-old baby develops tremors in his limbs and head, a twitching tongue, and involuntary jerking movements of his arms and legs.
- A 2-year-old child exhibits severe language and social delay and receives a diagnosis of autism.
- A 30-month-old boy, after receiving nitrous oxide anesthesia, begins exhibiting bizarre behaviors, regresses developmentally, and is diagnosed as autistic six months later.
- A 7-year-old boy is extremely clumsy, exhibits obsessive-compulsive behaviors, and has difficulty concentrating.
- A 7-year-old girl needs to attend a special kindergarten for handicapped children because she has an IQ of 60.
- A 12-year-old boy slowly loses his ability to walk and write.

cent becomes depressed and irritable, re-
, and starts skipping school.

n't concentrate or understand her instructors
her first semester of college.

oman becomes severely depressed and tries to
kill he

- A 28-year-old woman is unable to conceive.
- A 33-year-old with severe postpartum depression has thoughts of harming her infant.

All these women and children have one thing in common: their doctors and other health-care providers failed to diagnose them quickly and accurately. As a result, they were labeled with a variety of disorders, including depression, anxiety, mental illness, chronic fatigue syndrome, developmental delay, autism, Asperger's syndrome, cerebral palsy, iron-deficiency anemia, and attention deficit disorder. But in reality, they all suffered from the same medical condition—vitamin B_{12} deficiency.

This is not a rare, exotic disease. In fact, students read about it in their textbooks during their first years of medical school. Medical journals from the early 1960s on contain case studies of children injured by B_{12} deficiency, and adult cases were described as far back as the late 19th century. Yet somehow, this information doesn't translate into real-life practice.

Instead, B_{12} deficiency is commonly overlooked and untreated across all age groups. Even at-risk and symptomatic patients rarely get tested, and those who do get a correct diagnosis typically receive it at a late stage, after permanent damage has occurred.

Why? Because the information doctors and other clinicians receive about B_{12} deficiency is insufficient and grossly outdated—especially in the fields of gynecology, obstetrics, and pediatrics. Remarkably, health-care institutions and governments worldwide have no B_{12} awareness programs to educate the public or health-care providers about this silent crippler.

3

For reasons explained in subsequent chapters, B$_{12}$ deficie
especially likely to go undiagnosed in children, pregnant wome
women of child-bearing age. This is tragic, because vitamin B$_{12}$ is
critical for the growing fetus, and the developing embryo is particularly susceptible to deficiency. Poor B$_{12}$ status in a pregnant woman
increases the risk that her child will have neural tube closure defects
or other serious neurological problems, and low B$_{12}$ in a nursing
mother can cause irreversible neurological damage to a child.

How common is B$_{12}$ deficiency?

The NHANES survey (National Health and Nutrition Exam
Surveys, 1999–2002) found that 3 percent of children under the
age of 4 in the United States had a vitamin B$_{12}$ deficiency, with
serum B$_{12}$ levels of less than 200 pg/mL (picograms per milliliter).
This translates into 1 in every 33 children, an alarming number
in itself—but in reality, the percentage of children at risk for B$_{12}$-
related problems is far higher. That's because this survey didn't look
for children whose B$_{12}$ levels were marginal or low—in the range of
serum B$_{12}$ 200–300 pg/mL. Marginal deficiencies are far more common than outright deficiency, and even a marginal deficiency can
cause problems in growth, development, speech, learning, behavior,
mood, and socialization. Moreover, many marginal deficiencies are
proven to be true B$_{12}$ deficiency when other sensitive tests are used
in conjunction with serum B$_{12}$ assays.

The survey also identified B$_{12}$ deficiency in 3 percent of people
aged 20–39, 4 percent of people aged 40–59, and 6 percent of
people age 70 and older.[1] It found marginal or low B$_{12}$ levels—the
range where people are commonly symptomatic and have neurological and/or psychiatric symptoms—in an additional 15 percent
of people between the ages of 20 and 59.

The picture is even worse in other parts of the world. Studies in
Latin America indicate that around 40 percent of children and adults
have either low B$_{12}$ or outright deficiency. Approximately 70 percent
of Kenyan school children are either low in B$_{12}$ or overtly deficient, as
are 80 percent of preschoolers and 70 percent of adults in India.

1 L. H. Allen, "How Common Is Vitamin B$_{12}$ Deficiency?" *American Journal of Clinical Nutrition* 89, no. 2 (2009): 693S–96S

It's not surprising to see high rates of B_{12} deficiency in developing countries where poverty is rampant, a poor food supply exists, and vegetarian diets are often common. But it's shocking that the NHANES survey showed that more than 18 percent of adults in the United States, including women of child-bearing age, are either low in B_{12} or overtly B_{12}-deficient.

The NHANES study isn't the only research to show high rates of B_{12} deficiency in the United States. A Tufts University study in 2000, which analyzed data from the large-scale Framingham Offspring Study, found that nearly 40 percent of participants between the ages of 26 and 83 had plasma B_{12} levels in the "low normal" range. Nearly 9 percent had outright deficiencies, and 16 percent exhibited near deficiency. Remarkably, low serum B_{12} was as common in younger participants as in the elderly.[2] T.S. Dharmarajan, an expert in B_{12} deficiency, estimates that approximately 25 percent of the US population is B_{12}-deficient.[3]

And there's more bad news, because rates of B_{12} deficiency in children and young adults in the United States are climbing. As we explain in greater depth in Chapter 2, a wide range of factors—from dietary trends to medical treatments—are creating new risks for both children and their parents.

By the way, while this book focuses on children and women of childbearing age, it's also important to note that seniors, including grandparents who might be caring for young children, are at high risk for B_{12} deficiency. More than 20 percent of people over 60 and 26 percent of people over 70 have a marginal or overt deficiency.[4, 5, 6]

2 Judy McBride, study cited in "B_{12} Deficiency May Be More Widespread Than Thought," Agricultural Research Service website, U.S. Department of Agriculture (August 2, 2000), www.ars.usda.gov/is/pr/2000/000802.htm.
3 T. S. Dharmarajan and E. P. Norkus, "Approaches to Vitamin B_{12} Deficiency. Early Treatment May Prevent Devastating Complications," *Postgraduate Medicine*, 110, no. 1 (July 2001): 99–105
4 L. C. Pennypacker et al., "High Prevalence of Cobalamin Deficiency in Elderly Outpatients," *Journal of the American Geriatric Society*, 40, no. 12 (December 1992): 1197–204.
5 T. S. Dharmarajan, G. U. Adiga, and E. P. Norkus, "Vitamin B_{12} Deficiency. Recognizing Subtle Symptoms in Older Adults," *Geriatrics* 58 (2003): 30–38.
6 S. P. Stabler, "Screening the Older Population for Cobalamin (Vitamin B_{12}) Deficiency," *Journal of the American Geriatric Society* 43, no. 11 (November 1995): 1290–97.

Falling through the cracks: the heartrending costs of missed diagnoses

The effects of B$_{12}$ deficiency can be devastating—and, if the problem is diagnosed too late, these effects can be irreversible. So you might expect that doctors routinely check for this problem when they see women suffering from depression, weakness, fatigue, dizziness, nerve pain or numbness, restless legs, mental illness, anemia, multiple-sclerosis-like symptoms, chronic fatigue, infertility, or other medical problems that could point to B$_{12}$ deficiency. You might also assume that doctors likewise screen children with developmental delay or regression, behavioral changes, seizures, failure to thrive, or learning disabilities to see if B$_{12}$ deficiency is to blame. And you might presume they routinely screen pregnant and breastfeeding women in general—especially if these women are symptomatic or have risk factors.

In most hospitals, doctor's offices, and government clinics, however, none of this happens. In reality, most doctors, nurses, and allied health-care providers fail to diagnose B$_{12}$ deficiency in women of childbearing age, pregnant women, and nursing mothers, and many of these women develop irreversible symptoms as a result. Absent testing, doctors routinely ascribe the symptoms of B$_{12}$ deficiency in children to attention deficit disorder, behavioral and developmental disabilities, autism, "failure to thrive," or other conditions. For these children, the results of a missed or delayed diagnosis can be catastrophic—and they can last a lifetime.

———

When doctors admitted 15-month-old Jacob to the hospital, he was dehydrated and comatose. His mom, Jenna, said that he'd developed normally until 8 months of age, when he became irritable and apathetic.

Jacob was pale, had minimal responses to pain, and very poor muscle tone. His weight and length were below the 3rd percentile, and his head circumference was above the 10th percentile. Jacob had macrocytic anemia (in which the red blood cells are very large) and was diagnosed with severe B$_{12}$ deficiency.

6

Jacob's mom, who'd been a vegetarian for several years, had breast-fed him. Jenna was not anemic or macrocytic, but her serum B_{12} was also low.

Both Jacob and Jenna were treated with B_{12}. Jacob's neurological response was prompt, and he continued to improve over the next few months. Within two months, his head circumference increased to 75th percentile. Formal testing four years later (at age 5) showed him to be functioning in the borderline range of intellectual ability.[7]

―――

Eight-month-old Michael was referred to specialists because of his unexplained anemia and developmental delay. Michael developed normally until 4 months of age, when he became lethargic and irritable. His mom, Julie, had exclusively breastfed him, because she was unsuccessful when she tried to introduce solids. Julie was not a vegetarian and ate a diet that included meat, fish, and other animal products.

Michael was unable to sit unsupported or lift his head when face down. His head lagged when he was pulled up to sit. He had involuntary movements and tremors in his upper limbs, overactive reflexes, and very low muscle tone. His eyes did not fix or follow, and he had an exaggerated startle response.

Michael's blood work showed macrocytic anemia and a very low serum B_{12}. His EEG was abnormal, showing diffuse slow-wave activity.

Julie was also found to have a B_{12} deficiency. She was slightly anemic but was not macrocytic.

Michael's response to B_{12} therapy was remarkable, with an improvement in head growth up to the 90th percentile, disappearance of arm movements, and enhanced development. However, at the age of 2½ years, he still exhibited language delays. And at 5 years of age, he had mild to borderline intellectual retardation.[8]

―――

7 S. M. Graham, O. M. Arvela, and G. A. Wise, "Long-Term Neurologic Consequences of Nutritional Vitamin B_{12} Deficiency in Infants," *Journal of Pediatrics* 121 (1992): 710–14.
8 Ibid.

While working on our first book about B_{12} deficiency, we heard many heartrending stories like these from mothers and fathers whose children developed symptoms due to low B_{12}. Some lucky children got help in time; but for others, the diagnosis came too late. As a result, these children, their mothers, and their families suffered terribly.

In this book you will learn of the enormous toll B_{12} deficiency takes on the lives of children and their parents, and about the tremendous financial costs it imposes on families, health-care systems, and society. The sum damage so inflicted is further compounded by the fact that all this suffering is eminently avoidable and manifestly unnecessary. It is a travesty that *anyone* be allowed to suffer the devastating consequences of B_{12} deficiency, but reckless failure to diagnose and treat this condition in pregnancy and in pediatric patients is an exceptionally grievous form of medical neglect and an appalling offense against women, children, and future generations. We wrote *Could It Be B₁₂? Pediatric Edition* to create awareness of this preventable illness and to end the B_{12} deficiency epidemic— once and for all.

You can be part of this effort by becoming informed and spreading this vital information about B_{12} deficiency via social networks and mommy groups. The best way for parents to protect themselves and their families is to understand the scope of this problem.

In the next chapter, you'll learn what cobalamin (or vitamin B_{12}) is, why we need it, and the critical role it plays in sustaining human life. In addition, you'll learn about risk factors that can make you or your child a target for the devastating but entirely preventable disorder of B_{12} deficiency.

2

What Vitamin B₁₂ Is, What It Does, and the Dangers of Being Deficient

To ensure that you and your child don't become victims of the epidemic of B_{12} deficiency, you need to know the facts about this dangerous threat. Unfortunately, very few people do.

When I speak with mothers and expectant mothers about the risks of B_{12} deficiency, I often hear comments like these:

"I can't be deficient. I take a prenatal vitamin every day."

"We eat good food, not junk. So I know we're okay."

"I eat meat and animal products, so I can't be low in B_{12}."

"The doctor says our health is perfect, so I'm not worried."

"I'm a vegetarian, but I get enough B_{12} through yeast, tempeh, and nori."

Sadly, all of these assumptions are wrong. In reality, you or your child can be B_{12} deficient even if you both eat well, take standard supplements, and have no current symptoms. To understand why—and to understand just how devastating a B_{12} deficiency can be—you need to know a little about what vitamins are, and why B_{12} is unique.

WHY VITAMIN B₁₂ IS DIFFERENT, AND WHAT IT MEANS TO YOU

Your body needs 13 different essential vitamins to power the chemical reactions that build your tissues and organs, transform food into energy, remove toxins, fight infections, repair damage, and allow your cells to communicate with each other. It can't make these vitamins by itself, so it depends on you to provide them by eating the right foods.

Some vitamins, like vitamin D, are fat-soluble vitamins, and your body can store them. Others, including the various B vitamins, are water soluble. These vitamins need to be "restocked" every day. If they aren't, your levels will eventually drop below the normal threshold. If your stores drop even more, you'll develop a full-fledged deficiency. And the more deficient you become, the more dangerous the consequences will be.

One of the water-soluble vitamins your body needs to replenish constantly is vitamin B$_{12}$. This is where the story gets interesting, because B$_{12}$ is very unusual in several ways—and these peculiarities can make it hard for you to get enough of this crucial nutrient.

First, B$_{12}$—the largest and most complex of all the vitamins—is the only vitamin that you can't obtain from plants. Plants don't need B$_{12}$, so they don't produce or store it. Nor can you get B$_{12}$ from sunlight, as you can vitamin D.

So where does B$_{12}$ come from? It's produced by bacteria and micro-organisms in the guts of animals. Only bacteria and archaea (single-cell organism) have the enzymes needed for its synthesis. Sometimes tiny amounts are present in plants, due to contamination from the soil, but they do not provide an adequate source of the vitamin. In fact, these contaminates are often B$_{12}$ *analogs* that our bodies can't turn into the active form, making them useless for us. To obtain B$_{12}$ from your diet, you need to eat meat, poultry, fish, eggs, dairy products, or foods fortified with B$_{12}$—or, if you don't eat these foods, you need to take proper supplements. Table 2.1 lists the best food sources of B$_{12}$.

Here's another quirk that sets B$_{12}$ apart from the other vitamins. It's fairly easy to get a plentiful supply of those other vitamins if you eat a good diet, and it's even easier if you take a supplement as well. However, even a diet high in B$_{12}$, augmented with a supplement, isn't sufficient for many people. In fact, while you need only a tiny amount of B$_{12}$ each day, it's still remarkably easy to become deficient in this nutrient. That's because to get from your mouth into your bloodstream, vitamin B$_{12}$ has to follow a long and complex pathway—much different from those of other vitamins—and a roadblock along any part of that pathway can interfere with its journey.

TABLE 2.1: FOOD SOURCES OF VITAMIN B$_{12}$

Food	Micrograms (mcg)
Clams (3 oz)	84 mcg
Liver (3 oz)	71 mcg
Fish, mackerel (3 oz)	16.2 mcg
Crab (3 oz)	9.8 mcg
Salmon, sockeye (3 oz)	4.8 mcg
Tuna fish (3 oz)	2.5 mcg
Beef, top sirloin (3 oz)	1.4 mcg
Milk (240 mL–8 oz)	1.2 mcg
Yogurt (8 oz)	1.1 mcg
Cheese, Swiss (1 oz)	0.9 mcg
Egg (1 whole)	0.36 mcg
Chicken, breast (3 oz)	0.3 mcg
Fortified cereals (1 cup) (cyanocobalamin)	1.7–6.0 mcg

Here's a simplified explanation of the B$_{12}$ metabolic pathway:

1. The vitamin B$_{12}$ in food is bound to animal proteins, and your body has to free it. To cleave B$_{12}$ from protein, your stomach contains specialized cells in its lining called *parietal cells* that secrete *hydrochloric acid* and an enzyme called *pepsin.*

2. Your stomach's parietal cells also produce *intrinsic factor* (IF), a critical protein that makes its way into your intestine to be available for a later step in the B$_{12}$ absorption pathway.

3. Next, other proteins called *R-binders* ferry the B$_{12}$ into your small intestine.

4. In the intestine, intrinsic factor is bound to the B$_{12}$ (with the help of enzymes called *pancreatic proteases*) and carries it to the last section of the small intestine, the ileum. The cells that

line the ileum contain receptors that grab onto the B$_{12}$-IF complex, pulling it into the bloodstream.

5. In the bloodstream, another protein, *transcobalamin II*, transports vitamin B$_{12}$ into the portal circulation (blood sent to the liver from the small intestine).

6. Transcobalamin II is degraded within a lysosome, and free B$_{12}$ is finally released into the cytoplasm, where it can be transformed into the active forms and coenzymes (methylcobalamin and adenosylcobalamin). This is facilitated by two properly functioning cellular enzymes (methionine synthase and methylmalonyl-CoA mutase).

You don't need to fully understand all of the above in order to realize that getting B$_{12}$ to the cells in your body is a complex process, and it's all too easy for something to go wrong along the way. And when it does, the resulting deficiency can be life-altering.

WHAT CAUSES B$_{12}$ DEFICIENCY?

There are many causes of vitamin B$_{12}$ deficiency. Here are the six most commonly identified:

- An inability to absorb B$_{12}$ (as described above)
- A diet deficient in B$_{12}$
- An autoimmune disorder
- A genetic defect
- Medications that hinder the body's ability to use B$_{12}$
- A secondary deficiency in a child, stemming from a maternal deficiency prior to conception, during pregnancy, or during nursing

You might already be familiar with one cause of B$_{12}$ deficiency: pernicious anemia. In this autoimmune disorder, the body fails to produce intrinsic factor and hydrochloric acid, rendering B$_{12}$ in the diet useless. Many people learn about this disorder in science class, making it the most well-known (but *not* the most common) cause of B$_{12}$ deficiency.

Consequences of Late Diagnosis and Absent Screening

One recent case we came across in the medical literature involved a breastfed baby born to a vegan mother who took a multivitamin during her second and third trimester but not while nursing. The baby's doctor hospitalized him after he failed to gain weight, developed feeding problems, became pale and sleepy, and exhibited hypotonia ("floppiness").

At the time the doctors admitted the baby, his weight, length, and head circumference were below the 3rd percentile. He also had an enlarged liver and spleen and exhibited significant developmental delays.

Testing revealed that the infant had an extremely low B_{12} level, as well as iron deficiency. Doctors immediately treated him with a blood transfusion, intramuscular vitamin B_{12} injections, and iron supplements. His anemia improved quickly, and over time he began achieving developmental milestones. However, doctors say, "his development was still retarded seven months after the start of therapy."[1]

In another journal article, doctors described a child born to a mother who had undiagnosed B_{12} deficiency stemming from gastric bypass surgery six years earlier. At 4 months of age, the child was developmentally delayed, had abnormal blood cells, and exhibited brain atrophy (shrinkage) on a CT scan. Treatment with B_{12} reversed the blood abnormalities and some of the neurologic symptoms, and the baby gained weight. Doctors reported, however, that at 16 months, "gross motor and speech developments are significantly delayed."[2]

1 S. Guez, et al, "Severe Vitamin B_{12} Deficiency in an Exclusively Breastfed 5-Month-Old Italian Infant Born to a Mother Receiving Multivitamin Supplementation during Pregnancy," *BMC Pediatr* 12 (June 2012): 85. DOI: 10.1186/1471-2431-12-85.
2 M. Y. Celiker and A. Chawla., "Congenital B_{12} Deficiency Following Maternal Gastric Bypass," *J Perinatol* 29, no. 9 (September 2009: 640-42. DOI: 10.1038/jp.2009.16.

A much more common cause of B$_{12}$ deficiency is a condition called *atrophic gastritis*, which is an inflammation and deterioration of the stomach lining. Atrophic gastritis reduces the secretion of the stomach acid needed to separate vitamin B$_{12}$ from protein. Proton-pump inhibitors, antacids, and other acid-reducing medications (H2 blockers) can make this problem worse. Atrophic gastritis is most common among people over the age of 50, but it can also occur in children and women during child-bearing years who have autoimmune pernicious anemia or who are infected with *helicobacter pylori* (or *H. pylori*; the bacteria associated with ulcers).

THE INCIDENCE OF *HELICOBACTER PYLORI*

H. pylori infection in the United States affects around 20 percent of people under the age of 40, and 50 percent of those over the age of 60. It is estimated that 50 percent of the world's population is infected with *H. pylori*, which is yet another reason B$_{12}$ deficiency is very common.[3]

B$_{12}$ deficiency also occurs frequently in vegans, vegetarians, and people eating macrobiotic diets. Over 80 percent of long-term vegans who fail to supplement their diets adequately with B$_{12}$, and over 50 percent of long-term vegetarians, show evidence suggestive of B$_{12}$ deficiency.[4,5] People with bulimia or anorexia nervosa are also at elevated risk of becoming deficient.

Additional high-risk groups include people of any age who undergo gastric bypass for weight loss or have partial or complete stomach resections for other reasons (such as ulcers or cancer). These people lose the cells that produce hydrochloric acid and intrinsic factor, both of which are required to metabolize B$_{12}$. Intestinal surgery involving partial or complete removal of the ileum

3 A. R. Sepulveda et al., "Atrophic gastritis," Medscape reference (September 27, 2012), http://emedicine.medscape.com/article/176036-overview.
4 M. G. Crane et al., "Cobalamin (CBL). Studies on Two Total Vegetarian (Vegan) Families," *Vegetarian Nutrition: An International Journal* 2, no. 3 (1998): 87–92.
5 L. Bissoli et al., "Effect of Vegetarian Diet on Homocysteine Levels," *Annals of Nutrition and Metabolism* 46, no. 2 (2002): 73–79.

will also cause B_{12} deficiency, because the receptors needed for the absorption of B_{12} are located in this area.

Gastrointestinal disorders such, as Crohn's disease, enteritis, "blind loop" syndrome, or celiac disease (gluten enteropathy), can interfere with B_{12} absorption even if it's broken down correctly by the body. So can alcohol and many medications, including drugs commonly used to manage gastroesophageal reflux disease (GERD), ulcers, and diabetes. The drug metformin (Glucophage), which many young women take for non-insulin-dependent diabetes or polycystic ovarian disease, impedes B_{12} absorption in the ileum and can cause deficiency over time.

Other risk factors for low B_{12} include chronic pancreatitis, advanced liver disease, and past or current chemotherapy or radiation therapy. Interestingly, doctors are identifying more and more cases of B_{12} deficiency caused by infection with fish tapeworm (a parasite people can acquire from eating sushi or undercooked fish). This parasite appears in North America and Europe, as well as in developing countries.

Finally, a variety of inborn errors of B_{12} metabolism and transport can interfere with B_{12} metabolism at any step along the pathway. Some of these inborn errors can lead to an early death if they aren't diagnosed quickly, while others remain hidden for years before causing severe symptoms.

WHAT PARENTS NEED TO KNOW

Here's a risk factor that might surprise you: exposure to nitrous oxide (laughing gas), either during surgery or dental procedures or through recreational drug abuse, can inactivate B_{12}. Anesthesiologists often use nitrous oxide in emergency cesarean sections, putting infants at risk for severe B_{12} deficiency during their most crucial developmental period. See Chapter 10 for much more on this subject.

Here is a summary of risk factors that can make you susceptible to B$_{12}$ deficiency. While anyone, at any age, can become B$_{12}$ deficient, these factors will significantly elevate your risk.

Risk factors for developing B$_{12}$ deficiency

- Vegan, vegetarian, and macrobiotic diets
- Gastric and/or intestinal surgery, including bariatric surgery for weight loss (gastric bypass)
- Use of antacids, H2 blockers, and proton-pump inhibitors (e.g., Prilosec, Nexium, Protonix)
- Use of metformin or related drugs for diabetes, polycystic ovarian disease, or other conditions
- Dental procedures, medical procedures, or surgeries involving nitrous oxide, or recreational use of this drug
- A history of eating disorders (anorexia or bulimia)
- A history of alcoholism
- A family history of autoimmune pernicious anemia
- Liver disease (e.g., hepatitis, cirrhosis)
- Chronic pancreatitis
- Crohn's disease, irritable bowel syndrome, celiac disease (gluten enteropathy), bacterial overgrowth of the small bowel, or any other gastrointestinal disease causing malabsorption syndromes
- A history of autoimmune disorders—especially thyroid disorders such as Hashimoto's thyroiditis, Graves' disease, adrenal insufficiency, or insulin-dependent diabetes mellitus
- Pregnancy and breastfeeding
- *Helicobacter pylori* infection

- Diphyllobothriasis, a parasitic infection that is acquired by eating raw or undercooked fish infected with the parasite *Diphyllobothrium latum* (fish tapeworm)

- Giardiasis, an infection caused by *Giardia lamblia* (a parasite that colonizes and reproduces in the small intestine)

- Chemotherapy or radiation treatment (past or present) Note: If women get pregnant after chemotherapy or radiation treatment, their children can also be at risk for a deficiency.

- HIV infection or AIDS

How B_{12} deficiency wreaks havoc on the body

Every cell in the human body needs vitamin B_{12} in order to function. In addition, this vitamin plays a key role in the metabolism of folate (another B vitamin), and serves as a cofactor for two vital enzymatic reactions. It's also involved in the formation of DNA—the molecular blueprint for making the substances that create and maintain your body. That's why a deficit can literally harm you from head to toe.

Often, B_{12} deficiency strikes the nervous system, damaging the soft fatty material called myelin that surrounds and protects nerve fibers. This damage, called *demyelination*, is like the fraying of an electrical wire's insulation. Demyelination can disrupt nerve impulses in any part of the body. That's why, as you'll see in the following chapters, it can cause a wide array of terrifying cognitive, emotional, and physical symptoms.

B_{12} deficiency also makes it hard for your body to produce the red blood cells that carry oxygen to every cell. As a result, you could develop anemia. If your anemia becomes severe enough over time, you might require blood transfusions. A serious deficiency disrupts the bone marrow, which doctors occasionally misdiagnosis as acute leukemia.

In women, blood abnormalities resulting from B_{12} deficiency can affect the lining of the uterus and cervix, causing cervical dysplasia (abnormal cervical cell appearance) that can be mistaken for a precancerous condition. But B_{12} deficiency doesn't just mimic cancer warning signs; it also puts you at higher risk for certain cancers. Autoimmune pernicious anemia, the classic form of vitamin B_{12} deficiency, is a strong risk factor for stomach cancer, and mounting evidence is linking deficient levels of B_{12} to breast cancer as well.[6,7]

Your immune system also suffers if B_{12} levels are too low because it can no longer produce enough disease-fighting white blood cells. Your gastrointestinal system takes a hit, as well, because your body can't make enough cells to replace your intestinal lining efficiently.

> **Absorbing, utilizing, and transferring B₁₂ into your cells is a complex process that can be interrupted by a variety of factors.**

At the same time, B_{12} deficiency causes a breakdown in a crucial metabolic pathway that detoxifies the potentially dangerous amino acid homocysteine. As homocysteine accumulates in your blood, it dramatically increases your risk of stroke, coronary artery disease, and blood clots. If you become pregnant, high homocysteine levels will also make you more vulnerable to preeclampsia, a potentially fatal pregnancy complication.

In short, vitamin B_{12} plays crucial roles in the health of every system and every cell in your body—and that's why a deficiency can be so devastating. In the following chapters, you'll learn about the horrific effects that B_{12} deficiency can have on a developing fetus, a child, or a mother.

---

6 K. Wu et al., "A Prospective Study on Folate, B_{12}, and Pyridoxal 5'-Phosphate (B6) and Breast Cancer," *Cancer Epidemiology, Biomarkers and Prevention* 8, no. 3 (1999): 209–17.
7 Sang-Woon Choi, "Vitamin B_{12} Deficiency: A New Risk Factor for Breast Cancer?" *Nutrition Reviews* 57, no. 8 (1999): 250–53.

SYSTEMS AFFECTED BY VITAMIN B$_{12}$ DEFICIENCY

- Neurological
- Hematologic (blood)
- Immunologic
- Vascular
- Gastrointestinal
- Musculoskeletal
- Genitourinary

3

Three More Actors in the B_{12} Play

So far, we've focused our attention on vitamin B_{12}, the main character in our story. But to fully understand the impact of vitamin B_{12} deficiency, you need to meet three more cast members in this drama: a vitamin, an amino acid, and a gene, all of which work closely with B_{12} to help the body function properly. In this chapter, we'll take a look at the roles all three of these characters play, but to do this we'll need to delve into some science. So bear with us, because this information could save your life or that of your child.

B_{12}'S BIG SISTER: FOLATE

Vitamin B_{12} has a sister: vitamin B_9, also known as *folate* or *folic acid*. Little sister B_{12} serves as a coenzyme in her big sister's work. In her supporting role, B_{12} (in a form called methyl-B_{12}) converts folic acid into active folate, the form our bodies can use (see Figure 3.1). When there is a deficiency of little sister B_{12}, this conversion can't happen and big sister folate can't do her job. And if she can't do her job, very bad things can happen at any age, even in the youngest of us.

> Throughout this book, B_{12} and cobalamin are used interchangeably.

The worst damage a folate deficiency can do occurs during pregnancy. Folate deficiency during the first several weeks after conception puts a developing baby at higher risk for neural tube defects, which we'll talk about in Chapter 4.

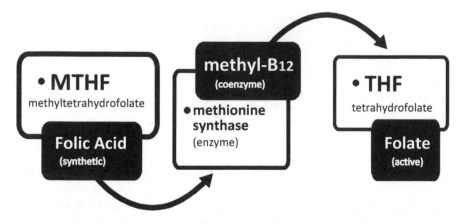

Figure 3.1. Folic acid is synthetic and not biologically active. It must be reduced to become metabolically active folate. This is accomplished through the actions of both the enzyme *methionine synthase* and the coenzyme *methylcobalamin*. Folate deficiency can result from a pure vitamin B$_{12}$ deficiency and/or an *MTHFR* genetic defect—in which the enzyme *methylenetetrahydrofolate reductase* is genetically mutated or faulty.

But a folate deficiency (either primary or stemming from low B$_{12}$ supplies) can damage a developing fetus, child, or adult in many other ways. That's because the development of *every human cell* depends on an adequate supply of folate, along with an adequate supply of vitamin B$_{12}$. Here are some of the important jobs of folate, which it can only do if "little sister" B$_{12}$ is around, too:

- It plays a crucial role in making and repairing DNA.

- It plays a key role in the methylation of genes—that is, the "turning on" or "turning off" of genes.

- It's involved in producing healthy red blood cells, preventing anemia during pregnancy.

- It's critical for rapid cell division and growth during pregnancy and infancy.

- It's involved in the creation of substances that allow the immune system to function optimally, protecting the body against cancer and other illnesses.

Because your body can't produce folic acid or folate on its own, you need to obtain it through your diet. Folic acid is water-soluble and synthetic, and it's used in fortified foods and most supplements, whereas folate is the naturally occurring form of the vitamin, found in many fruits, vegetables, beans, and other plant foods. Folate is particularly abundant in dark green leafy vegetables like spinach. (In fact, the terms *folate* and *folic acid* come from the Latin word *folium*, meaning leaf.)

Table 3.1 shows the best sources of folate. But remember that no matter how many folate- or folic-acid-rich foods you include in your diet, *these nutrients can't do their job without enough B₁₂.*

TABLE 3.1: SOURCES OF FOLATE (VITAMIN B₉)

Food	mcg
Beef liver, braised, 3 oz	215
Black-eyed peas, ½ cup	105
Asparagus, boiled, 4 spears	89
Lettuce, romaine, 1 cup	64
Avocado, ½ cup	59
Spinach, 1 cup	58
Broccoli, ½ cup	52
Green peas, ½ cup	47
Kidney beans, ½ cup	46
Peanuts, dry roasted, 1 oz	41
Wheat germ, 2 tablespoons	40
Tomato juice, canned, ¾ cup	36
Orange, fresh, 1 small	29
Papaya, ½ cup	27
Banana, 1 medium	24

HOMOCYSTEINE: THE GOOD GUY WHO TURNS BAD

As you saw in the last section, B$_9$, our first supporting character in the B$_{12}$ drama, is a hero (as long as you get enough of it). With the help of its little sister B$_{12}$, it helps to keep every cell in your body strong and healthy.

The next character in the B$_{12}$ story, however, starts out as a hero but often turns into a villain. And when it switches from good guy to bad guy, it puts people of any age—including infants and children—at risk for deadly vascular problems. This character is *homocysteine*.

WHAT IS HOMOCYSTEINE AND WHY IS IT SO BAD FOR YOU?

The story of homocysteine begins with the food you eat. Overall, your food contains 20 amino acids (or proteins), one of which is *methionine*. Your body breaks down methionine into smaller particles. One of these is a molecule called *s-adenosylmethionine* (or SAMe for short). SAMe, in turn, breaks down into even smaller substances, one of which is homocysteine. When everything's working right, your body quickly recycles homocysteine back into methionine with the help of vitamin B$_{12}$ and folate (see Figure 3.2).

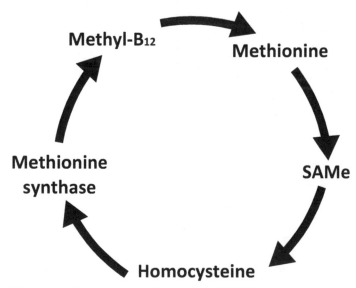

Figure 3.2. Homocysteine is continuously being converted back into methionine in the presence of active B$_{12}$ (methylcobalamin).

Any excess homocysteine winds up in your liver, which breaks it down with the help of vitamins B_{12}, B_6, and folate.

So far, so good. But here's the catch. If you're deficient in any one of these B vitamins, this normal cycle breaks down and homocysteine accumulates in your blood, with no place to go (see Figure 3.3).

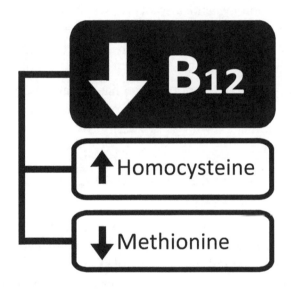

Figure 3.3. When B_{12} deficiency is present, homocysteine will rise and methionine will decrease.

That's dangerous, because homocysteine is a bad guy when left on its own. Excess homocysteine causes your blood vessels to become less elastic, making it harder for them to dilate, and damages their inner lining. That damage, in turn, allows cholesterol, collagen, and calcium to attach to the inner walls of your blood vessels, where they can form sticky deposits called atherosclerotic plaques. These plaques narrow your arteries and drastically increase your risk of suffering deadly disorders such as coronary artery disease, heart attacks, strokes, deep vein thromboses, pulmonary embolisms, carotid and renal artery stenosis (narrowing), or aneurysms (ballooning of damaged blood vessels). In addition, elevated homocysteine levels alter your biochemistry in ways that appear to promote abnormal blood clotting.[1]

In addition, elevated homocysteine causes pregnancy complications. These include placental abruption, recurrent pregnancy loss, intrauterine growth restriction, and neural tube defects. Furthermore, homocysteine also decreases the production of nitric oxide[2]—a substance crucial to healthy blood vessel function. Decreased nitric oxide, in turn, is strongly linked to both atherosclerosis and high blood pressure.

Five to 10 percent of the population has elevated homocysteine levels,[3] and one primary cause of the problem is a low level of folate and/or vitamin B$_{12}$. (Low levels of vitamin B$_6$ also contribute, but to a lesser degree.)

Why folate alone can't protect you against high homocysteine

Doctors are now well aware of the dangers of high homocysteine and the benefits of folic acid therapy. Unfortunately, few of these doctors fully understand the critical role that vitamin B$_{12}$ plays in detoxifying homocysteine. This is a serious oversight, because people with high homocysteine levels often respond fully only when they're given large amounts of B$_{12}$ as well.

Why? As we mentioned earlier in the chapter, *people who are deficient in B$_{12}$ can't assimilate folic acid properly*. As a result, much of the folic acid gets trapped in an inaccessible form. That's why testing for B$_{12}$ deficiency—and delivering treatment, if a deficiency is detected—must always be part of a homocysteine-lowering program.

1 O. Nygard et al., "Plasma Homocysteine Levels and Mortality in Patients with Coronary Artery Disease," *New England Journal of Medicine* 337 (1997): 230–36.
2 Nitric oxide, by the way, should not be confused with the anesthetic agent nitrous oxide. The two names sound alike, but there is no relationship.
3 J. D. Kark et al., "Plasma Homocysteine and Parental Myocardial Infarction in Young Adults in Jerusalem," *Circulation* 105, no. 23 (2002): 2725–29.

MTHFR: A GENE THAT CAN SPELL BIG TROUBLE FOR MOM AND BABY

With two of the cast members in our B_{12} drama out of the way, it's time to zero in on the final one. This bad guy is a mutation in a gene called methylenetetrahydrofolate reductase or *MTHFR*.[4]

You have two copies of the *MTHFR* gene, one from each parent. Unfortunately, there's a good chance that you don't have two *good* copies. Overall, 40 percent of Americans have one defective *MTHFR* gene and 10 percent have two defective genes.[5] If you have one copy of the defective gene, you're a carrier of *MTHFR* deficiency. If you have two copies, you have a *MTHFR* deficiency. Why does this matter? Because *MTHFR* deficiency can put both you and your child at risk for serious or even fatal health problems.

WHY *MTHFR* DEFICIENCY PUTS YOU AND YOUR CHILD IN DANGER

Normally, the *MTHFR* gene produces plentiful amounts of the important enzyme called *methylenetetrahydrofolate reductase* (also abbreviated MTHFR). However, a defective copy of the gene produces smaller amounts of this enzyme. That's a big problem, because your body needs the enzyme to convert inactive forms of B_{12} and B_9 into the necessary active forms (see Figure 3.4).

There are two common mutations of the *MTHFR* gene, designated as C677T and A1298C. People with *MTHFR* deficiency resulting from one mutated copy of each gene (C677T and A1298C)—that is, people who are *compound heterozygous*—have a reduced ability to convert inactive forms of B_{12} and B_9 into active forms; this condition is associated with increased plasma homocysteine levels. For people with two mutated copies of the C677T gene—that is, people who are *homozygous*—the effects are thought to be far greater, resulting in increased risk of thrombosis. Research is conflicting regarding the A1298C gene mutation. However, heterozygotes of either C677T or

4 The *MTHFR* gene provides instructions for making an enzyme called methylenetetrahydrofolate reductase (MTHFR). This enzyme plays a role in processing amino acids, and is critical for a chemical reaction involving forms of B_9. MTHFR (in no italics) is the enzyme and *MTHFR* (in italics) denotes the gene.
5 "MTHFR Deficiency," www.counsyl.com/diseases/mthfr-deficiency.

A1298C (single mutation carriers) may have intermediate levels of enzyme activity but no increase in plasma homocysteine levels.

So if you have two C677T mutations—or one defective copy of each gene (C677T and A1298C)—you're at higher risk of being deficient in B_{12} and B_9. And that can put your unborn child at risk for neural tube defects, or even cause a miscarriage, especially if combined with other B_{12}-deficiency risk factors.

The MTHFR enzyme also plays a crucial role in converting the amino acid homocysteine—that "good guy, bad guy" chemical we just talked about—into methionine. So MTHFR deficiency leads

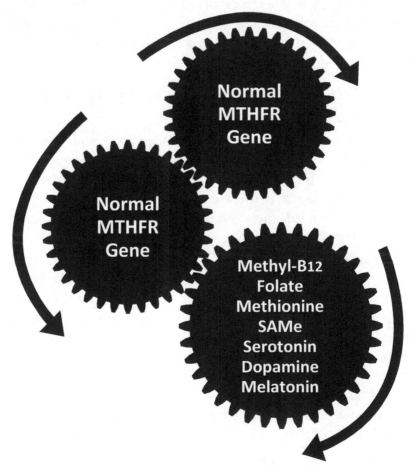

Figure 3.4. When the *MTHFR* gene is normal, the body can properly convert inactive B_{12} and folic acid into the active forms, thereby producing other critical biological substances (e.g., neurotransmitters).

not only to elevated levels of homocysteine, but also to low levels of methionine, which is a big problem. That's because methionine does a lot of important things for your body. Here are some of them:

- It processes fats in the liver.

- It's necessary for the production of glutathione, which is a very important detoxifier and antioxidant.

- It's a building block of s-adenosylmethionine (SAMe). SAMe helps your body create and break down the brain chemicals dopamine, serotonin, and melatonin, and it's also crucial for a healthy immune system.

For methionine to play all of these roles, it needs to be available in plentiful supply in your body. If an MTHFR defect lowers levels of methionine, the scientific literature indicates that you or your child will be at increased risk for cancer, stroke, heart problems, congenital defects, depression, miscarriages, fatty liver disease, migraines, and chemical sensitivities. MTHFR defects have also been associated with an increased incidence of autism.[6]

It's important to know that people with an MTHFR defect can actually have high serum B_{12} and B_9 levels. That's because their bodies have a problem converting the inactive forms into the active forms. The B_{12} and B_9 they have are therefore fictitious, causing misleading results on certain blood tests (e.g., serum B_{12}).

WHAT PARENTS NEED TO KNOW

So how can you protect yourself against this stealthy villain? You can't change a defective gene, but you can help it do its job better. In Chapter 11, we'll talk about how to find out if you have defective copies of the *MTHFR* gene, and we'll explain how to compensate if you do, by ensuring that you get sufficient quantities of active B_{12} and folate through your diet and supplements.

---

6 M. Boris et al., "Association of *MTHFR* Gene Variants with Autism," *Journal of American Physicians and Surgeons* 9, no. 4 (winter 2004): 106–8.

Putting it all together

Metabolic Substances & Pathways Utilizing B_{12}	B_{12} Needed For	B_{12} Helps Make These Neurotransmitters
• methionine	• methionine cycle	• serotonin
• SAMe	• protein synthesis	• dopamine
• homocysteine	• folate cycle	• epinephrine
• betaine	• purine synthesis	• norepinephrine
• choline	• trans-sulfuration	
• DNA	• RNA synthesis	
• DNA methylation	• DNA synthesis	
• folate		
• thymidine synthesis		
• dUMP		
• DTMP		

Figure 3.5. Vitamin B_{12} is involved in numerous metabolic pathways and is needed to create vital substances for health and life. A deficiency interrupts an array of normal metabolic cycles and conversions, thereby creating disease.

As Figure 3.5 suggests, in the circle of life, everything is interconnected. One small genetic error, one defective enzyme, or a shortage of one vitamin can interrupt critical metabolic processes, causing disease or even death. But when you're knowledgeable about all of the processes involved in B_{12} metabolism and how they can go wrong, you can take active steps to protect yourself.

And now that you're familiar with the three additional players in the B_{12} drama, it's time to get back to our main character: vitamin B_{12} itself. In the next chapter, we'll look at the time period in which B_{12} deficiency does its greatest damage: during pregnancy and nursing.

4

The Risks and Dangers of Low B₁₂ When You're Pregnant or Nursing

If you're pregnant or planning to conceive, you already know that eating the right foods is crucial to your baby's health. And it's especially critical during the first few weeks of pregnancy, when every system in your baby's body is rapidly developing.

But suppose you do have good eating habits and plenty of access to healthful food. Could you still have a nutritional deficiency that is wreaking havoc on your unborn? One that is causing injury, disability, or potentially even death? The answer is yes, when it comes to vitamin B_{12}.

WHY PREGNANCY IS A HIGH-RISK TIME FOR B₁₂ DEFICIENCY

When you're pregnant, your baby is totally dependent on you for a good supply of B_{12}. Your body sets aside a store of B_{12} and its "big sister" folate in the placenta, and your unborn baby can use this B_{12}—but it can't make or synthesize B_{12} on its own. So if you're low in B_{12}, your baby is low, too.[1]

And here's another twist to the story. Even if you have adequate stores of B_{12} in your body, your unborn baby can still suffer if you fail to take in enough B_{12} in your diet. That's because only *newly absorbed vitamin B_{12} readily crosses the placenta*. So most of the vitamin B_{12} that your body stockpiled earlier is off-limits to your baby.[2]

1 A. M. Molloy et el., "Effects of Folate and Vitamin B_{12} Deficiencies during Pregnancy on Fetal, Infant, and Child Development," *Food and Nutrition Bulletin* 29, no. 2 suppl. (June 2008): S101–11; discussion S112–15.
2 J. R. Davis, J. Goldenring, and B. H. Lubin, "Nutritional Vitamin B_{12} Deficiency in Infants," *American Journal of Diseases of Children* 135 (1981): 566–67.

Also, the concentration of B$_{12}$ in your blood drops during the course of your pregnancy for a variety of reasons. These reasons include hormonal changes, increased dilution of the blood, changes in the concentration of B$_{12}$ binding proteins, and placental transport of B$_{12}$ to the fetus. B$_{12}$ levels reach their lowest point at 32 weeks of pregnancy and then appear to increase right before delivery, reaching a "normal" level after birth.[3]

Add in other risk factors—for instance, the *MTHFR* gene defect we talked about in Chapter 3 or the risk factors we outlined in Chapter 2—and there's a significant chance that your unborn baby could have low B$_{12}$ levels. And that risk is even greater for one particular group of women who think they're eating right for their baby.

A CRUEL IRONY

Babies who are B$_{12}$-deficient as a result of their moms' deficiency often become anorectic and reject solid foods. This leads their mothers to breastfeed them even longer and further worsen their B$_{12}$ deficiency.

ONE BIG RISK FACTOR: HOW VEGETARIAN AND VEGAN DIETS INCREASE YOUR RISK

There are many reasons why women (and, as a result, their babies) can be low in B$_{12}$. But one of the most common causes is a maternal diet that doesn't include animal products.

This isn't a criticism of meat-free diets, which tend to be very healthful because they're high in phytochemicals and antioxidants and generally low in artificial colorings and additives. If these diets contain plenty of supplemental B$_{12}$, they can protect you against

3 H. Van Sande et al., "Vitamin B$_{12}$ in Pregnancy: Maternal and Fetal/Neonatal Effects—a Review. *Open Journal of Obstetrics and Gynecology* 3, no. 7 (2013), 599–602. Article ID: 37330, DOI: 10.4236/ojog.2013.37107.

cancer, heart disease, and diabetes. But if they don't, they can harm or even kill an unborn baby.

Because B_{12} occurs naturally only in animal products, a vegan diet, which excludes eggs and dairy products as well as meat, fish, and shellfish, provides virtually no natural B_{12}. A lacto-ovo-vegetarian diet, while it can include eggs and cheese, may provide too little B_{12}, especially if a woman has followed this diet for several years or longer. Even a macrobiotic diet, which excludes most animal protein with the exception of fish, can lead to B_{12} depletion. And the risk of B_{12} deficiency grows exponentially if a mother who's eating a vegetarian, vegan, or macrobiotic diet has any of the other risk factors we outlined in Chapter 2.

> A mother following a meat-free diet may have "normal" vitamin B_{12} levels, but her child is still at risk of a B_{12} deficiency.

Many pregnant women eating a meat-free diet think they're safe from a B_{12} deficiency because they're taking supplements. However, many vegetarians and vegans take supplements that are ineffective or even harmful (see Chapter 11 for details), which is particularly dangerous during pregnancy.

RISKS OF MEAT-FREE DIETS WHILE BREASTFEEDING

All of these factors put the babies of mothers following meat-free diets at higher risk of B_{12} deficiency. And that risk, unfortunately, becomes even greater when these mothers breastfeed. Research indicates that vegetarian and vegan mothers often breastfeed for long periods of time, meaning that their infants could be getting a B_{12}-deficient diet for many months after birth.

What's more, children of mothers eating meat-free diets can be severely crippled by B_{12} deficiency even if their breastfeeding mothers have "normal" B_{12} levels. That's because, just as in the case of pregnancy, the mother's body will not mobilize existing stores of B_{12} efficiently in order to make up for a dietary deficiency. "Consequently," hematologist Julian Davis and his colleagues say, "even mothers who have only recently become vegans and who have no hematologic or biochemical evidence of vitamin B_{12} deficiency may place their nurslings at risk for this vitamin deficiency."[4]

Mothers who follow vegetarian, vegan, or macrobiotic diets are devastated and feel tremendous guilt when their children suffer harm due to B_{12} deficiency, but nearly all of these tragedies are the fault of a health-care system that fails to screen pregnant and nursing mothers for low B_{12} and to educate them about this critical vitamin. In addition, these mothers are often misled by an array of misinformation in different books and websites regarding B_{12} and the vegetarian diet. In reality, these mothers—just like their children—are innocent victims.

NO GUARANTEES—NO MATTER WHAT YOU EAT

If you eat meat and dairy, or supplement a meat-free diet correctly, you'll greatly reduce your risk of developing a B_{12} deficiency that can harm your unborn baby. However, that doesn't necessarily mean that you're out of the woods. As we noted in Chapter 2, there are many risk factors for B_{12} deficiency, and doctors rarely screen patients with these risk factors for low B_{12}. As a result, millions of women around the world are unknowingly putting their babies at risk.

A recent study, in fact, showed that one third of infants develop elevated methylmalonic acid (MMA) levels by 6 weeks of age. (As we'll explain in Chapter 11, elevated MMA levels are a sign of inadequate levels of B_{12}.) The key thing to know about this study is that it involved mothers eating non-vegetarian diets. The researchers who conducted the study report: "Even in this population we found biochemical evidence of cobalamin [B_{12}] deficiency."[5] This indicates, they say, that doctors underestimate the prevalence of low B_{12} in newborns.

4 J. R. Davis, J. Goldenring, and B. H. Lubin, "Nutritional Vitamin B_{12} Deficiency in Infants," *American Journal of Diseases of Children* 135 (1981): 566–67.
5 A.-L. Bjorke Monsen et al., "Determinants of Cobalamin Status in Newborns," *Pediatrics* 108, no. 3 (2001): 624–30.

That's a huge mistake, because—as we'll show in this chapter and the next—a missed diagnosis of B_{12} deficiency during pregnancy, in the neonatal period, or during nursing can have devastating lifelong consequences for both mother and baby. And sometimes, those consequences can be fatal.

———

Thirty-eight-year-old Monica, desperate for a child, kept trying despite her four early miscarriages. Eventually, her doctor tested her to see if a MTHFR defect might be interfering with her ability to carry a pregnancy. Monica indeed had the MTHFR C677T genotype defect, and more testing showed elevated homocysteine. Her doctor admitted

---

KEY FACTS ABOUT MATERNAL B_{12} DEFICIENCY

- Adequate B_{12} status during pregnancy is critical because maternal B_{12} deficiency endangers both mother and child.

- Not all moms with B_{12} deficiency develop symptoms.

- Anemia and macrocytosis (enlarged red blood cells) do not always occur in B_{12} deficiency. Doctors who rule out B_{12} deficiency because blood cells appear normal will miss many cases of maternal B_{12} deficiency.

- When anemia is present in pregnancy, doctors often assume the anemia is caused by iron or folate deficiency without checking for low B_{12} as a potential culprit.

- B_{12} and folate deficiency are known to cause macrocytosis, and both can cause anemia. Prenatal vitamins, which contain high doses of folic acid, will mask this effect by reducing the red cell size and improving the anemia. Physicians who mistakenly wait for these signs will therefore miss an ongoing B_{12} deficiency, endangering both mother and fetus.

he was surprised to find that while Monica's folate was normal, she was severely B$_{12}$ deficient (B$_{12}$ < 150 pg/mL). A bone marrow biopsy showed evidence of moderate megaloblastosis, caused by her B$_{12}$ deficiency.

Monica began injectable B$_{12}$ therapy, and within two months her homocysteine was normal. Best of all, she completed a successful pregnancy soon afterward.[6]

HOW LOW B$_{12}$ IN PREGNANCY DAMAGES A BABY'S BRAIN AND BODY

In the next chapter, we'll describe the tragic symptoms that occur in infants with B$_{12}$ deficiency. For now, however, we're going to focus on the unseen damage that can be occurring to a B$_{12}$-deficient baby in the womb, even if mom feels totally fine.

LOW B$_{12}$ AND NEURAL TUBE DEFECTS

Neural tube defects (NTDs) are abnormal openings in the brain or spinal cord that can lead to severe disability or death. NTDs are one of the most common birth defects, affecting more than 300,000 children each year.[7]

The two most common defects are *spina bifida* and *anencephaly*. In spina bifida, the spinal column fails to close completely. This typically results in nerve damage leading to at least some paralysis of the legs. In anencephaly, a major area of the brain and skull fails to develop. Babies with anencephaly are either stillborn or die shortly after birth.

Most women know that low folic acid is a risk factor for NTDs. And the medical community is acutely aware of this issue, which is why many governments now fortify cereals and other foods

6 M. Candito, et al., "Clinical B$_{12}$ Deficiency in One Case of Recurrent Spontaneous Pregnancy Loss," *Clinical Chemistry and Lab Medicine* 41, no. 8 (August 2003): 1026–27.
7 National Center on Birth Defects and Developmental Disabilities, *Neural Tube Defects (Annual Report)*, U.S. Centers for Disease Control and Prevention (2012).

with folic acid. But as we explained in Chapter 3, *folic acid can't do its job without enough B_{12}*. So doctors who focus solely on telling women to take folic acid are still leaving these women at high risk for a secondary folate deficiency due to low B_{12}. And that, in turn, puts their children at high risk for NTDs. Here's what the research shows:

- A 2009 study reported in the journal *Pediatrics* found that women with vitamin B_{12} deficiency in early pregnancy were up to *five times more likely* to have a child with NTDs, such as spina bifida, than women with high levels of B_{12}.[8]

- Another study in the *American Journal of Clinical Nutrition* found a three-fold increase in the risk of NTDs in mothers who had vitamin B_{12} status in the lowest quartile, regardless of folic acid fortification. The study concluded that vitamin B_{12} fortification in conjunction with folic acid supplementation may reduce NTDs more effectively than folic acid fortification alone.[9]

Clearly, doctors are helping pregnant women, or those who want to conceive, by educating them about the importance of getting enough folic acid or folate—but they're actively harming these same women by failing to inform them that folic acid (B_9) can't protect them and their children unless a plentiful amount of little sister B_{12} is along for the ride.

OTHER DAMAGE THAT LOW B_{12} IN *UTERO* CAN CAUSE

In addition to putting babies at risk for NTDs, low B_{12} *in utero* can cause a wide range of other problems affecting every system in a developing fetus's body. Here's a list of problems that the scientific literature links to maternal B_{12} deficiency, either alone or in combination with a folic-acid deficiency, during pregnancy:

8 A. M. Molloy et al., "Maternal Vitamin B_{12} Status and Risk of Neural Tube Defects in a Population with High Neural Tube Defect Prevalence and No Folic Acid Fortification," *Pediatrics* 123 (2009): 917–23.
9 M. D. Thompson et al., "Vitamin B_{12} and Neural Tube Defects: The Canadian Experience," *American Journal of Clinical Nutrition* 89 Suppl. (2009): 697S–701S.

Problems linked to inadequate B$_{12}$ & B$_9$ intake before conception and in the early weeks of pregnancy

- Congenital malformations
- NTDs
- Congenital heart defects
- Cleft lips
- Limb defects
- Urinary tract anomalies
- Preterm delivery
- Low birth weight
- Fetal growth retardation
- Elevated homocysteine
- Spontaneous abortion
- Placental abruption

And adequate B$_{12}$ isn't just necessary *during* pregnancy; it's also necessary for a pregnancy to occur in the first place. In the absence of adequate B$_{12}$, it's difficult for immature eggs to mature, for fertilized eggs to implant, and for a healthy placenta to develop.

———

Gina, who was 33 and had been married for seven years, couldn't understand why she couldn't get pregnant. She also was experiencing progressive weakness and had difficulty walking. In addition, she noticed that she had a poor memory.

Gina's doctors drew a blank until her lab work finally showed macrocytic anemia. At that point, she received a referral to a hematology clinic. There, doctors diagnosed her with B$_{12}$ deficiency and started her on injections of the vitamin.

Within three months, Gina felt far better mentally and her gait vastly improved. And within six months, she became pregnant. Her long years of waiting for a child ended when she delivered a healthy baby girl.[10]

———

Linda, a 32-year-old infertile woman, underwent four rounds of artificial insemination without success before her doctors detected both iron deficiency and vitamin B$_{12}$ deficiency. They began treatment with oral iron and injected vitamin B$_{12}$, and within two months, Linda became pregnant. She now has two healthy children, the second conceived without any need for fertility treatments.[11]

———

WHY LOW B$_{12}$ DURING PREGNANCY ENDANGERS MOM AS WELL

So far we've discussed how low B$_{12}$ can endanger an unborn child. However, a deficiency also puts mothers at risk—both during pregnancy and afterward.

Research indicates that low B$_{12}$ increases a mother's risk of pre-eclampsia. In this condition, pregnant women develop high blood pressure, facial and leg swelling, abdominal pain, severe headaches, and other symptoms. If preeclampsia continues, it can turn into eclampsia—a condition that is life-threatening.

In addition, one study links low maternal B$_{12}$ during pregnancy to an increased risk for gestational diabetes. This study also found that women with B$_{12}$ deficiency who developed gestational diabetes during pregnancy were more likely to gain weight and become insulin resistant in the years following delivery.[12]

10 Y. Menachem, A. M. Cohen, and M. Mittelman, "Cobalamin Deficiency and Infertility," *American Journal of Hematology* 46, no. 2 (1994): 152.
11 J. Sanfilippo and Y. Liu, "Vitamin B$_{12}$ Deficiency and Infertility: Report of a Case," *International Journal of Fertility* 36, no. 1 (1991): 36–38.
12 P. Saravanan and C. S. Yajnik, "Role of Maternal Vitamin B$_{12}$ on the Metabolic Health of the Offspring: A Contributor to the Diabetes Epidemic?" *British Journal of Diabetes and Vascular Disease* 10 (2010): 109–14.

B$_{12}$ DEFICIENCY IN PREGNANCY: WHY ARE DOCTORS SILENT?

If you're pregnant or hoping to conceive, your doctor will go to great lengths to tell you about many dangers to avoid. You'll hear about the risks of smoking or drinking alcohol during pregnancy, and about the dangers of contracting contagious diseases like the flu. You'll also get lectures on avoiding junk food and any unnecessary medications—and you'll be well versed on taking folic acid or B$_9$.

However, as we mentioned earlier, most medical professionals receive virtually no accurate information or training about the effects of B$_{12}$ deficiency on a developing fetus. Textbooks for nursing students usually don't cover this issue at all, while textbooks for medical school students and practicing physicians offer only a few paragraphs. And what little information there is in these books is grossly out of date, despite the wealth of ongoing published research.

As a result, obstetricians, pediatricians, and other health professionals mistakenly believe that B$_{12}$ deficiency is extremely rare. But in fact, it's one of the most common risks a pregnant woman and her child face—and it's entirely preventable.

WHAT PARENTS NEED TO KNOW

Because your own doctor isn't likely to be aware of how dangerous (and common) B$_{12}$ deficiency is during pregnancy, it's up to you to make sure that you and your child are safe. In Chapter 11, you'll learn steps you can take to prevent a B$_{12}$ deficiency during pregnancy, get information on how to get tested to make sure you're not low in B$_{12}$, and find out how a knowledgeable doctor can treat any existing deficiency quickly and effectively.

5

Vitamin B$_{12}$ Deficiency in Infants and Toddlers

In the last chapter, we told you how B$_{12}$ deficiency can injure or even kill an unborn child or its mother. However, the dangers of B$_{12}$ deficiency don't end there. In fact, they're just beginning. That's because your beautiful baby—even if he or she looks perfectly normal—may have a silent B$_{12}$ deficiency. And there's a strong chance that your doctor has never checked your child for this possibility, or checked *you* to see if you're deficient. This could therefore threaten your baby's health, especially if you breastfeed without correcting the problem.

> "My baby became symptomatic, not me. The result was irreversible brain damage in my breastfed child."
>
> —a B$_{12}$-deficient mother

But what if you don't breastfeed, or you supplement your breast milk with formula? You may think that this guarantees your baby's safety, but it doesn't. That's because the amount of B$_{12}$ in formula isn't enough to treat an existing deficiency.

To understand this, picture the body's vitamin B$_{12}$ supply as a glass of water. If the glass is full, and only a little water is lost each day, you can refill the glass with a few drops from the faucet. But if the glass is half empty—or almost completely empty—you'll need much more water to refill it.

Similarly, a child with a high B$_{12}$ level needs just a little bit of B$_{12}$ each day to stay healthy. But a child with very low levels needs a lot of B$_{12}$ to catch up. So while a child who receives formula may not die of a B$_{12}$ deficiency, he or she may still suffer the neurological effects of chronic low B$_{12}$.

To make matters worse, months can go by without your doctor recognizing the signs, symptoms, or risk factors of B$_{12}$ deficiency at your child's well-baby visits. In fact, your pediatrician may not contemplate B$_{12}$ deficiency even when severe symptoms are present.

———

George's mom Mary, a vegan for five years, had a normal, uneventful pregnancy. She breastfed her son up to the age of 14 months, and then introduced vegetables and fruits.

George stopped developing normally when he reached the age of 6 months. Concerned, his doctors ordered physical and stimulation therapy, but it didn't help. Months passed, and Mary became more and more alarmed as George grew weaker and lost his ability to smile and look at her. When he was 18 months old, his doctor admitted him to the hospital with a diagnosis of "psychomotor retardation."

Blood tests showed that George was anemic and had enlarged red blood cells. His doctors also found that he had severely delayed motor milestones and abnormal muscle tone. He had poor head control, exaggerated muscle stretch reflexes, slow "blink" reflexes, and little reaction to noise and light. He couldn't fix his eyes on objects, and he had trouble swallowing. However, his body weight, length, and head circumference were normal for 18 months of age.

Examining George's eyes, doctors found partial optic atrophy (a wasting away of the optic nerve). His EEG revealed a general slowing of brain waves, a very abnormal finding. A brain CT scan revealed diffuse atrophy, meaning that George's brain had shrunk.

George's doctors finally diagnosed severe B$_{12}$ deficiency, which was due to his mother's diet, and immediately started George on daily injections of B$_{12}$. He improved dramatically, and his apathy and poor muscle tone disappeared within hours. After five weeks of B$_{12}$ therapy, George's spontaneous motor activity and visual behavior were normal, and so was his EEG.

Eight months after aggressive B₁₂ therapy, George's brain CT was normal, showing that his diffuse brain atrophy had reversed. But George, who was 26 months old at this point, still had big problems. According to his doctors, he functioned at a 12-month-old level. He was just beginning to walk and had a vocabulary of only five words. And he still exhibited abnormal reflexes, muscle stiffness, spasticity, and some involuntary rhythmic muscular contractions and relaxations.

Happy ending? Not really. Granted, George did not die, did not wind up in a permanent coma, and was not completely physically disabled. But George will most likely have lifelong cognitive problems and sensory-motor disabilities—all of which could have been prevented if Mary's doctors had screened her for B₁₂ deficiency during pregnancy and breastfeeding, and instructed her on the need to supplement a vegan diet with correct forms of B₁₂.[1]

—

THE LIFE-THREATENING COSTS OF LOW B₁₂ IN INFANTS AND TODDLERS

As infants and young children grow and learn, they rapidly master new skills such as rolling, crawling, walking, and talking. As evidenced by George's story, children with B₁₂ deficiency—which damages the cells in the brain and nervous system—fall further and further behind in reaching these developmental milestones. Worse yet, B₁₂ deficiency is progressive and can quickly lead to irreversible damage early in life. Infants are more vulnerable than adults to permanent brain injury because their nervous systems are still developing.

Prevention as well as screening are needed to protect children from the spectrum of neurological injury that B₁₂ deficiency can cause during this time of rapid growth and development. Early diagnosis and treatment may completely or partially reverse

1 K. Stollhoff and F. J. Schulte. "Vitamin B₁₂ and Brain Development," *European Journal of Pediatrics* 146 (1987):201–5.

symptoms, but there's a very brief window (as described immediately below) before time runs out.[2,3]

In adults, symptoms of B$_{12}$ deficiency often develop slowly. If an adult's B$_{12}$ stores initially are adequate, it can take a few years for problems to become significant. But infants who are born to mothers with B$_{12}$ deficiency, and who are exclusively breastfed, can be deficient at birth or develop a deficiency within the first few months of life. Infants who are breastfed appear to be most vulnerable for B$_{12}$ deficiency when they are between the ages of 4 and 12 months.[4,5]

——

Frantic, Tracy brought her son Samuel into the emergency department. Samuel, 8 months old, was critically ill.

Until he reached 4 months of age, Samuel had developed normally. Then he became irritable and increasingly lethargic. Tracy tried to introduce solids into his diet, but he refused to eat them. So Tracy, who wasn't a vegan or vegetarian, exclusively breastfed him.

A few weeks earlier, Samuel had become irritable, rejecting even breast milk. He began to sleep more and more, and became weak and "floppy."

Examination in the emergency department revealed that Samuel's eyes did not fix or follow, and he had an exaggerated startle response. Samuel was unable to sit unsupported or lift his head when placed on his abdomen, and his head lagged when he was pulled up to a sitting position. He also exhibited rhythmic snakelike movements in his upper limbs. He had very poor muscle tone, and his reflexes were hyperactive.

2 S. M. Graham et al., "Long-Term Neurologic Consequences of Nutritional Vitamin B$_{12}$ Deficiency in Infants," *Journal of Pediatrics* 121, no. 5, part 1 (November 1992): 710–4.
3 S. A. Rasmussen, P. M. Fernhoff, and K. S. Scanlon, "Vitamin B$_{12}$ Deficiency in Children and Adolescents," *Journal of Pediatrics* 138, no. 1 (2001): 10–17.
4 R. Muhammad et al., "Neurologic Impairment in Children Associated with Maternal Dietary Deficiency of Cobalamin—Georgia, 2001," *Morbidity and Mortality Weekly Report* 52, no. 4 (January 31, 2003): 61–64).
5 M. M. Black, "Effects of Vitamin B$_{12}$ and Folate Deficiency on Brain Development in Children," *Food and Nutrition Bulletin*, 29, no. 2 suppl. (June 2008): S126–S31.

Samuel's blood work showed severe B_{12} deficiency and anemia. His EEG showed diffuse slow-wave brain activity, and a CT scan revealed severe brain atrophy.

When Samuel received injectable B_{12}, his doctors saw "remarkable" results. His head growth reached the 90th percentile and the snakelike movements in his extremities disappeared. In addition, he began to make progress developmentally. However, at 30 months of age, he had significant language delay. And when he was 5 years old, tests showed that he had "mild to borderline intellectual retardation."[6]

If doctors had screened Samuel and his mother routinely and pre-scribed high-dose B_{12} or given B_{12} injections during pregnancy and nursing, he would not have a lifelong intellectual disability. An ounce of prevention is worth a pound of cure—especially when a child's life and future are at stake.

———

Over time, B_{12} deficiency causes failure to thrive—eventually, it can lead to coma or even death. A paper published in the October 2005 issue of *Public Health Dietitian* cited several serious cases of infant B_{12} deficiency in the authors' geographic area, one resulting in the death of a baby.[7] Yet despite a wealth of similar published medical articles, no guidelines or standard-of-care changes have been developed and implemented to prevent this treatable but crippling and deadly disorder.

If doctors catch B_{12} deficiency in time, they can correct it quickly, and affected infants and toddlers could regain all of their skills and possibly make a full recovery. Sadly, however, many cases aren't diagnosed until children become permanently intellectually disabled. And many children with chronic low or marginal B_{12} levels are never diagnosed at all.

6 S. M. Graham et al., "Long-Term Neurologic Consequences of Nutritional Vitamin B_{12} Deficiency in Infants." *Journal of Pediatrics* 121, no. 5, part 1 (November 1992): 710–4.
7 M. Van Oeveren, "Vitamin B_{12} for Vegan Mothers and Their Babies," *Public Health Dietitian* (October 2005): 1–13.

If B$_{12}$ deficiency goes unrecognized in infancy, treating the disorder later at the toddler stage can lead to rapid improvement. However, some areas of the brain may be permanently injured, giving rise to fine-motor problems, lower IQ, speech and language deficits, developmental delay, and behavioral problems. Here's how one pediatric neurologist put it: "Infantile vitamin B$_{12}$ deficiency may cause lasting neurodisability, even though vitamin B$_{12}$ supplementation leads to rapid resolution of cerebral atrophy and EEG abnormality."[8] The extent of recovery depends on the age at which the B$_{12}$ deficiency began, the severity of the deficiency, how long it was present, and at what age treatment was started.

TIME IS BRAIN

The phrase "time is brain" emphasizes that tissue of the human nervous system is quickly lost as a stroke progresses, and that rapid evaluation and therapy are crucial. This phrase also applies to children with B$_{12}$ deficiency because lack of B$_{12}$ in the rapidly growing brain can cause permanent injury and lifelong disabilities if not recognized early. Each day, week, and month a child's brain is starved of B$_{12}$ results in progressively poorer outcomes. Time is of the essence! In addition, progressive B$_{12}$ deficiency can further injure children's brains by causing strokes due to hyperhomocystinemia.

SIGNS AND SYMPTOMS OF LOW B$_{12}$ IN THE EARLY MONTHS AND YEARS

B$_{12}$ deficiency is a great masquerader, and pediatricians often misdiagnose its symptoms or overlook them entirely. For example, doctors may mistake the irritability or gastric symptoms of B$_{12}$ deficiency for colic or gastroenteritis. In addition, they might mistake an apathetic or dull infant for an "easy" or "good" baby. And moms

8 U. von Schenck et al., "Persistence of Neurological Damage Induced by Dietary Vitamin B$_{12}$ Deficiency in Infancy. *Archives of Disease in Childhood* 77 (1997): 137–9.

can be fooled too, especially when doctors reassure them that nothing serious is wrong.

Sometimes, infants develop symptoms rapidly, becoming severely ill over the course of just a few weeks. Other times, the symptoms of B$_{12}$ deficiency aren't obvious at first. Older infants and young toddlers typically show developmental delay or regression, slowly revealing their symptoms over time. This may lead doctors to opt for "waiting and watching," or to misdiagnose the child with autism (see Chapter 8). Some infants may also receive a diagnosis of cerebral palsy because of their poor muscle tone. But no matter how B$_{12}$ deficiency presents itself, doctors rarely diagnose the problem correctly at the outset.

———

Megan started showing signs of developmental delay at 6 months of age. Her doctors, uneducated about B$_{12}$ deficiency, decided to "wait and watch," thinking that she might have some form of cerebral palsy, perhaps develop autism, or simply outgrow her problems.

As the months passed, Megan continued to miss developmental milestones and continually grew weaker. Over the next seven months, she kept falling further behind.

When Megan was 13 months old, her pediatrician referred her to a pediatric developmental specialist who ordered more tests. An MRI showed brain atrophy, a classic sign of B$_{12}$ deficiency in infants. A urinary organic acid profile showed grossly elevated methylmalonic acid, and blood work revealed a severely low serum B$_{12}$.

Despite aggressive B$_{12}$ therapy, Megan will never fully recover. Her brain and nervous system are permanently injured, and she will most likely require lifelong care. At 2 years and 7 months of age, she cannot walk or talk, and has seizures. She is babbling and cruises while holding onto furniture, which places her developmentally at around 9 months of age.

Megan's devastating symptoms occurred because her mother had an undiagnosed B$_{12}$ deficiency and breastfed her. Megan's mom was *not a vegetarian, but suffered from a B$_{12}$ deficiency that her OB/GYN never caught. Megan's mom told us that she herself was asymptomatic, which was remarkable given that she too had very low B$_{12}$ levels. This is why screening pregnant and nursing moms is critical.*[9]

———

Babies and toddlers affected by severe B$_{12}$ deficiency begin to lose their speech and social skills, and they become apathetic and irritable. They often refuse to eat, and they regress to the point where they can no longer sit, crawl, stand, or walk. Often their heads and bodies grow too slowly, and they fail to gain weight, becoming thin and weak. (However, this is not always the case. George, whose story we reported earlier, had a normal body weight, length, and head circumference for his age despite his severe deficiency.) Brain scans frequently show atrophy (shrinkage) of the cerebral cortex.

Two common symptoms in infants and young children with B$_{12}$ deficiency are abnormal arm or leg movements and seizures. One study of 15 infants and young children with neurological symptoms due to B$_{12}$ deficiency found that 7 had seizures and 5 had tremors.[10] The mean age of the children was 11.7 months, and all 15 had "neurodevelopmental retardation" and poor muscle tone.

The type, severity, and duration of involuntary movements related to B$_{12}$ deficiency can vary. Abnormal movements include tremor (involuntary shaking), chorea (brief, irregular muscle contractions that sometimes appear snakelike), and myoclonus (jerking). Abnormal movements may be the first symptom a parent or doctor spots, or they may occur after treatment starts.

Sometimes abnormal movements result from a combination of tremors and myoclonus and can be misinterpreted as seizures or convulsions. In other cases, however, a child's abnormal movements truly do stem from seizures. And some children, as the following case shows, may have both tremors and seizures.

9 This child's story was communicated to the authors personally by her mother.
10 F. Incecik, S. Altunbaşak, G. Leblebisatan, "Neurologic Findings of Nutritional Vitamin B$_{12}$ Deficiency in Children," *Turkish Journal of Pediatrics* 52, no. 1 (January–February 2010): 17–21.

———

First-time mom Katie breastfed her daughter Alicia. The first two months of Alicia's life were unremarkable. At the age of 3 months, however, she developed a fine tremor. At 4 months of age, she began having generalized tonic-clonic (grand mal) seizures. Alicia's pediatrician treated her with the antiseizure drug phenobarbital and also administered a single dose of pyridoxine (vitamin B6), but her seizures continued. She underwent lumbar puncture (spinal tap) and routine blood work. Her blood work showed anemia, but all other results were normal.

A week later, Alicia was admitted to the hospital for excessive sleepiness and therapy-resistant seizures. Doctors also noted her small head and body size. Her body weight and length were still in the normal range, but had both significantly decreased from 75th percentile at birth to the 3rd percentile.

Alicia had very poor muscle tone and was lethargic. An MRI revealed severe brain shrinkage, and her repeat blood work showed macrocytic anemia. Her serum B_{12} was very low, and her methylmalonic acid and homocysteine were markedly elevated.

Doctors immediately started therapy with injectable B_{12}, and within 24 hours, Alicia's seizures ceased. She became more awake and responded to stimuli. Her head circumference normalized within four months. Laboratory values were all normal at follow-up, but her development was delayed.

Alicia's mom, Katie, was not a vegetarian and was not symptomatic for B_{12} deficiency. However, further testing showed that she too was indeed B_{12} deficient, despite her lack of symptoms. Additional tests revealed that Katie had autoimmune pernicious anemia, and she is now on lifelong injectable B_{12} therapy.

Alicia's doctors followed up on her case, and reported that she started walking independently at the age of 19 months. However, she spoke only a few simple words at age 3. By the age of 7, she was attending a special kindergarten for disabled children and showed "moderate mental retardation."[11]

———

As the cases in this chapter show, doctors often fail to diagnose B$_{12}$ deficiency quickly in infants and children. That's why it's important for parents and medical professionals to be vigilant—and for parents to insist on testing any symptomatic child, even if doctors are resistant.

A child with B$_{12}$ deficiency or low B$_{12}$ may have some or many of the following signs and symptoms. If your own infant or child exhibits any of these symptoms, find a doctor who will conduct thorough B$_{12}$ testing. Do not take "no" for an answer.

While standing up to your pediatrician might be difficult and very stressful, the stakes are too high for you to give in. So stand your ground and find a new doctor if your current pediatrician does not agree to follow the testing guidelines we outline in Chapter 11. Days count when an infant or young child has a B$_{12}$ deficiency, and early treatment can mean the difference between a normal life and permanent disability or death.

11 G. C. Korenke et al., "Severe Encephalopathy with Epilepsy in an Infant Caused by Subclinical Maternal Pernicious Anaemia: Case Report and Review of the Literature," *European Journal of Pediatrics* 163, no. 4–5 (April 2004): 196–201.

SIGNS AND SYMPTOMS OF B₁₂ DEFICIENCY IN INFANTS AND TODDLERS

- Drowsiness or lethargy
- Poor interaction
- Irritability
- Weakness
- Poor muscle tone (hypotonia)
- Vomiting
- Poor suckling/poor appetite
- Uncontrollable involuntary movements—tremors, chorea, myoclonus
- Seizures
- Poor weight gain
- Poor head growth
- Failure to meet developmental milestones (smiling, rolling over, babbling, lifting head, sitting, standing, walking)
- Problems with speech and swallowing
- Poor coordination of movement
- Unsteady walk with poor balance
- Failure to thrive
- Anemia
- Macrocytosis
- Language/speech delay
- Developmental delay or regression
- Lower IQ
- Mental retardation/intellectual disabilities
- Symptoms resembling autism or a diagnosis of autism (see Chapter 8)

6

Signs and Symptoms of Low B_{12} in Preteens and Adolescents: From Subtle to Deadly

As you've seen, harrowing symptoms can develop within months or even weeks in infants and young children with B_{12} deficiency. However, the picture is often very different for older children and teens. Many B_{12}-deficient older children and adolescents have symptoms too subtle for doctors or even parents to pick up. In particular, their mental symptoms—memory deficits, slight declines in fluid IQ,[1] fatigue, mood changes, attention problems, or depression—may be written off as behavior problems, "growing pains," or academic issues.

In some cases, however, the problems seen in children and teens become dramatic, as a deficiency begins causing overt neurological symptoms too pronounced to ignore. Signs of advancing disease can range from muscle weakness to paralysis, psychiatric disorders, or even blindness. In one horrifying case reported several years ago, a 13-year-old boy was only weeks away from death when doctors finally identified his B_{12} deficiency.[2]

That teen, by the way, wasn't a vegan or vegetarian. And this illustrates an important point: While children eating vegan or vegetarian diets are the most likely to have low B_{12} levels, they aren't the only young people prone to develop a deficiency. The same risk factors that apply to adults apply to children of any age. Here is a list of them.

1 Fluid IQ is the ability to think logically and solve problems in new and unfamiliar situations, or the ability to reason quickly and think abstractly. It is necessary for all logical problem solving (e.g., scientific, mathematical, and technical).
2 Michele Mandel, "Boy Paralyzed by 'Forgotten Disease,' " *Toronto Sun* (December 17, 2007).

Risk Factors for B$_{12}$ Deficiency in Children and Teens

- Gastrointestinal
  - Atrophic gastritis
  - Crohn's disease
  - Celiac disease (gluten enteropathy)
  - Stomach or ileal surgery
  - Pancreatic insufficiency
  - Abnormal ileal receptor (Imerslund-Gräsbeck disease)
  - Proton-pump inhibitor and/or H2-blocker use
  - *H. pylori* (the bacteria that cause ulcers)
  - Giardiasis (a common parasitic disease)
  - Diphyllobothriasis (fish tapeworm)
- A vegan, vegetarian, or macrobiotic diet
- Eating disorders (bulimia, anorexia)
- Autoimmune disorders (e.g., pernicious anemia, thyroid, Addison's disease, vitiligo)
- Family history of pernicious anemia
- Exposure to nitrous oxide via dental/medical procedures or recreational abuse

While children or teens with any of these red flags are at risk, parents of children following a vegan, vegetarian, or macrobiotic diet need to be especially vigilant. Parents whose children follow these diets need to find doctors who can counsel them about supplementing properly, and who will test their children's serum B$_{12}$ and urinary MMA levels regularly. As Joel Fuhrman, a physician and a practicing vegetarian, says: "It is entirely irresponsible for a health professional not to recommend B$_{12}$ supplementation in some form or frequent monitoring of MMA . . . for those who do not consume any animal products in their diets. No controversy exists."[3]

3 Fuhrman's quote appears on www.breathing.com/articles/vitamin-b12-vegan.htm.

Portraits of deficiency

No matter what type of diet your child eats, if his or her medical history includes any of the risk factors listed, it's crucial to ask for testing. That's because B_{12} deficiency can affect every aspect of a child's life, and it can lead to permanent damage if not caught early.

Here's a look at some of the most common ways this deficiency can affect your child:

"I'm so tired . . ."

In the preteen and teen years, it's common for kids to loll around, act lazy, and sleep in. But children with anemia due to B_{12} deficiency aren't just being lazy. Instead, they're very sick.

Anemia can stem from a deficiency of iron, vitamin B_{12}, and/or folate. The type of anemia that often results from B_{12} and folate deficiency is called *megaloblastic* anemia. In this type of anemia, the bone marrow produces unusually large red blood cells that can't mature. Because these cells don't work properly, they can't carry enough oxygen to other cells throughout the body. This leaves people fatigued, pale, weak, and lightheaded. Megaloblastic anemia affects physical growth, thinking, behavior, mood, and overall health, making it difficult or impossible for children or teens to keep up academically, socially, or athletically. And if teens get pregnant, it can severely affect both their health and their baby's.

Most doctors mistakenly believe that megaloblastic anemia is an early symptom of B_{12} deficiency, but it actually tends to be a late-stage symptom. The neurological signs and symptoms of B_{12} deficiency commonly precede the hematologic (blood) signs. The next case illustrates that by the time anemia occurs, B_{12} deficiency is often transitioning from debilitating to dangerous—and the neurological damage that accompanies the anemia is often progressing from temporary to permanent.

When 14-year-old Sasha came to the ER, her doctors immediately knew that she was in serious trouble. She had paraplegia (paralysis), ataxia (severely impaired coordination), extreme fatigue, and a fever. Her symptoms, which began a few months earlier, had rapidly progressed over the past three weeks.

Sasha's lab test confirmed vitamin B$_{12}$ deficiency and macrocytic anemia, and her brain MRI showed atrophy. Her fever workup eventually led to a diagnosis of tuberculosis, and more tests revealed that the tuberculosis had involved the terminal ileum, resulting in her B$_{12}$ deficiency.

Doctors treated Sasha aggressively and report that she responded well. Ten months after her treatment began, she was able to eat, write, and speak normally, as well as walk and ride a bicycle. However, she does have some degree of "foot drop"—an inability to lift the front of her feet when she walks. This is a direct result of B$_{12}$ deficiency attacking the myelin surrounding her nerve cells.[4]

———

"SCHOOL IS SO HARD. I JUST CAN'T DO IT!"

Millions of children and teens find school a struggle because they have learning disorders. Often, there's no way to know what causes these problems. But in many cases, the hidden culprit is low B$_{12}$.

Research on children eating vegan diets shows that low B$_{12}$ in childhood can dramatically impair their ability to learn. Worse yet, learning problems can persist even when children begin obtaining adequate amounts of B$_{12}$ from their diets. For instance, in 1985, Dr. Wija van Staveren and colleagues began following a group of infants being raised on vegan diets. Testing the children in their early years, the researchers noticed subtle but significant impairments in the psychomotor functioning of vegan children as compared to those eating meat and dairy products.

Told of these findings, many parents of the vegan children participating in the study chose to switch their children to diets containing

4 T. D. Toosi et al., "Neuropathy Caused by B$_{12}$ Deficiency in a Patient with Ileal Tuberculosis: A Case Report," *Journal of Medical Case Reports* 2 (March 21, 2008): 90. DOI: 10.1186/1752-1947-2-90.

milk, eggs, and in some cases meat. On average, the children began eating animal products at around the age of 6. When the children reached adolescence, the researchers again compared them to a group of children raised from birth on diets that included animal products. Each of the 48 formerly vegan children and the 24 control children took a 90-minute battery of tests that measured their cognitive skills, and the researchers measured their serum B_{12} and methylmalonic acid levels.

Many of the children raised until age 6 on vegan diets were still B_{12} deficient, even after years of eating at least some animal proteins. "We found a significant association between cobalamin [B_{12}] status and performance on tests measuring fluid intelligence, spatial ability, and short-term memory," Staveren and colleagues reported, with the formerly vegan children scoring lower than the control group members in each case.[5]

> Children with B_{12} deficiency need higher-than-normal amounts of the vitamin in order to replenish their depleted stores.

The deficit in the early vegan children's fluid intelligence is particularly troubling, the researchers say, "because it involves reasoning, the capacity to solve complex problems, abstract thinking ability, and the ability to learn. Any defect in this area may have far-reaching consequences for individual functioning."

Most of the children switched from vegan diets had B_{12} intakes close to the Recommended Dietary Allowance at the time of the follow-up study, yet many of them continued to suffer from B_{12} deficiency. "Because these subjects consumed a diet extremely low in cobalamin [B_{12}] from birth up to the age of six years," the researchers speculated, "their cobalamin stores may never have reached an optimal level and moderate intakes may not have been sufficient for obtaining normal serum cobalamin status."[6]

5 M. Louwman et al., "Signs of Impaired Cognitive Function in Adolescents with Marginal Cobalamin Status," *American Journal of Clinical Nutrition* 72 (2000): 762–69.
6 It's puzzling that although the parents of the children in this study were highly educated, and researchers detected the children's low B_{12} status in infancy, a number of these children's personal physicians apparently did not conduct regular B_{12} testing during   57

If your child has a learning disability that stems from low B$_{12}$, it's critical to identify the problem early on, because if you don't, things may get far, far worse. Stay vigilant!

WHAT PARENTS NEED TO KNOW

One crucial take-away lesson from this research is that if your child becomes B$_{12}$-deficient, simply switching him or her to a diet higher in B$_{12}$ and offering a multivitamin supplement is not enough. Children with B$_{12}$ deficiency need higher-than-normal amounts of the vitamin in order to replenish their depleted stores, just as adults do, and the standard vitamin formulas that parents typically buy are not up to the job. So if your child turns out to be deficient in B$_{12}$, insist on proper supplementation.

Seven-year-old Tommy had always appeared to be a typical healthy, happy boy. But now he was in the hospital, with doctors working hard to uncover the cause of his alarming symptoms.

Tommy's problems had started a few months earlier. He'd begun engaging in obsessive-compulsive behaviors, including climbing the stairs over and over and lining up his toys. In addition, he had increasing trouble concentrating, making it hard for him to learn.

Over time, his gait became progressively unsteady, and his clumsiness progressed to intermittent falling. Because his symptoms came on so slowly, his parents didn't notice them until several family members and friends pointed them out.

At the hospital, doctors found that Tommy exhibited acute cerebellar ataxia—an unsteady gait that typically stems from cerebellar

---

childhood, or provide B$_{12}$ injections when needed—the only likely explanation for the children's continuing deficiency. We would consider this to be substandard or negligent medical care for children with identified deficiencies.

disease or injury. His weight and body mass index were below the 3rd percentile, and the doctor's examination showed clear signs of neurological dysfunction. His parents told the doctor that Tommy and the rest of the family followed a vegan diet.

Lab tests showed that Tommy was anemic and macrocytic. His eventual diagnosis: subacute combined degeneration of the spinal cord, meaning that some areas in Tommy's brain, spinal cord, and peripheral nerves were injured.

After two months of B₁₂ therapy and initial extensive nutritional counseling, Tommy's neurological symptoms had nearly resolved. His doctors reported that his cognition was "improved," but only time will tell if his learning problems persist.[7]

What is subacute combined degeneration (SCD)?

Subacute combined degeneration is a disorder of the spinal cord, brain, and nerves caused by prolonged vitamin B₁₂ deficiency. Symptoms of SCD include abnormal sensations (parasthesias), clumsiness, stiff or awkward movements, weakness, mental problems, and visual difficulties. SCD predominantly affects the spinal cord, but also affects the brain and the peripheral (body) nerves, which is the reason for the term *combined*.

In SCD, the myelin sheath covering the nerves becomes damaged. As a result, a person's ability to sense pressure, vibration, and touch becomes diminished. Eventually, the entire nerve cell is affected, potentially causing permanent sensory, motor, or cognitive disabilities.[8]

---

7 J. R. Crawford and D. Say, "Vitamin B₁₂ Deficiency Presenting as Acute Ataxia," *British Medical Journal Case Reports* (2013). DOI:10.1136/bcr-2013-008840.

8 B. Katri and D. Koontz, "Disorders of the Peripheral Nerves," in *Bradley's Neurology in Clinical Practice*, 6th ed., ed. R. B. Daroff et al. (Philadelphia: Elsevier Saunders, 2012): chapter 76.

"My body feels weird."

The neurological damage caused by low B$_{12}$ often creates odd sensations far away from the brain and spinal column. For instance, it's common for people to feel tingling sensations or "pins-and-needles" feelings in their hands or feet.

———

Five-year-old Lilly kept flapping her hands sideways as if to get something sticky off them. She would also do this with her feet. She complained to her mom that her hands and feet felt "funny"—like they were burning.

Lilly had been taking a proton-pump inhibitor most of her life, starting in infancy. Because proton-pump inhibitor use is a risk factor for B$_{12}$ deficiency, we the authors instructed her mom to get Lilly tested.

Sure enough, the little girl had an elevated urinary methylmalonic acid level, indicating B$_{12}$ deficiency. And once she began receiving treatment for that deficiency, her symptoms disappeared.

———

"I'm scared, mom. i think i'm losing my mind."

In Chapter 9, you'll see that B$_{12}$ deficiency can cause mental symptoms ranging from mild anxiety or depression to outright psychosis. For now, we want to point out that older children and teens with low B$_{12}$ are particularly susceptible to automatically receiving a diagnosis of mental illness from their doctors, because problems like depression, suicidal thinking, severe anxiety, and schizophrenia often begin to appear in the high school and early college years.

As a result, it's easy for a doctor to prescribe antidepressants, antianxiety drugs, or antipsychotic drugs without looking for the root cause of a child's symptoms. The result: the B$_{12}$ deficiency worsens, and so do mental symptoms. But if a doctor catches the problem early enough, these symptoms can be reversible.

——

Sixteen-year-old Michael was irritable and apathetic. He wept frequently, became anxious when he was separated from his mother, and complained of vague pains. Over the course of a year, his symptoms grew progressively worse. He couldn't sleep, didn't eat well, and regressed behaviorally. He started skipping school, grew less and less talkative, and became more and more isolated from his peers.

Michael was frequently agitated and spent far too much time in front of his computer. He also ran up big debts on his parent's credit cards buying items online.

Michael's family was mystified. They described him as formerly extroverted, happy, and active. He'd never exhibited any signs of mental illness, and there was no history of it in his family. He didn't do drugs, and he'd been well liked in school.

Eventually, Michael developed even scarier symptoms. He started having auditory and visual hallucinations, and he began thinking that other people were looking at and talking about him. He developed delusions of guilt, believing that he had sinned and would be punished. And he believed that his thoughts were being broadcast so that others could hear them.

Michael's mother took him to a doctor who found that Michael had poor memory skills and impaired attention and concentration. The doctor also noted that Michael had suicidal thoughts. Michael's judgment, abstract thinking, and grasp on reality were impaired. His thought processes were sluggish, his voice was soft, and he showed little emotion.

Psychological testing revealed that Michael had severe anxiety. A physical exam showed that he had poor balance, his shoulders were rigid, and he exhibited cogwheel rigidity in his left elbow (a jerky "ratcheting" motion when the doctor moved the arm). He had poor coordination, was unable to keep his balance with his eyes closed, and didn't swing his arms normally when he walked. He also had a mask-like expression, and his tongue was inflamed.

Luckily, Michael's doctor ordered extensive lab tests—and he was smart enough to check for B$_{12}$ deficiency, even though Michael wasn't a vegetarian or a vegan. As it turned out, Michael was indeed B$_{12}$-deficient as a result of an infection with H. pylori *in his stomach. Michael was mildly anemic, but not macrocytic. His doctor's diagnosis: "Mood disorder with mixed psychotic features due to vitamin B$_{12}$ deficiency."*

Michael began B$_{12}$ therapy along with treatment for his H. pylori *infection. His neurological symptoms resolved and his behavior became more normal as well. His doctor followed up with him monthly for another six months and reported that he suffered no further psychiatric symptoms.[9]*

DISTURBING WARNING SIGNS FOR PARENTS OF TEENS

As you can see from the case studies in this chapter, vitamin B$_{12}$ deficiency can mimic the symptoms of anything from attention problems to learning disabilities to depression to autism to schizophrenia. So it's crucial for doctors to ask: Are there hundreds of thousands of children taking stimulants, antianxiety drugs, antidepressants, or antipsychotics when low B$_{12}$ is actually the real culprit in their cases? And could we give these children an opportunity for full, healthy lives simply by providing simple, safe, inexpensive B$_{12}$ treatment?

And here is another, even darker question we need to ask. Given the link between B$_{12}$ deficiency and mental illness, could low B$_{12}$ play a role in some school shootings? Obviously, there are many reasons for these horrific events, and low B$_{12}$ is just one possibility. But many school shooters have a background of mental illness, learning disability, attention deficits, autistic symptoms, or social isolation. Add low B$_{12}$ or an overt deficiency into the equation, and

9 A. E. Tufan et al., "Mood Disorder with Mixed, Psychotic Features Due to Vitamin B$_{12}$ Deficiency in an Adolescent: Case Report," *Child and Adolescent Psychiatry and Mental Health* 6 (2012): 25. www.capmh.com/content/6/1/25

this may be the last straw that pushes some marginally functional children over the edge. In fact, severe B_{12} deficiency may even be the *sole* factor in some children's suicidal and homicidal behavior.

And consider the following as well: Many older children and teens abuse nitrous oxide, which inactivates B_{12} (see Chapter 10), or they receive this drug during medical or dental procedures, putting them at even higher risk for a B_{12} deficiency, and altering their thinking and behavior in dangerous or deadly ways.

Right now, we don't know how many older children and teens are struggling to get by in school and in life while bearing the heavy burden of low B_{12} or B_{12} deficiency. That's because while more and more researchers are studying the devastating effects of B_{12} deficiency in adults and seniors, few are looking at its effects on younger people. And as the cases in this chapter show, that's a tragic mistake.

Because there is such a knowledge deficit in this area, *it is up to you as a parent to be alert* and to identify any potential signs of B_{12} deficiency in your child. Below is a list of the warning signs to look for in an older child or teen. If you see any of them, insist on thorough testing. Also, remember that children (just like adults) can undergo drastic neurological deterioration even when standard blood tests show no signs of traditional B_{12}-deficiency anemia. So don't rely on tests for anemia or a serum B_{12} test alone. (See Chapter 11 for information on the right tests to get.)

Signs and Symptoms of Low B$_{12}$ in School-Aged Children and Teens

- Depression
- Apathy
- Suicidal or homicidal thoughts
- Changes in behavior
- Mental illness
- Paranoia
- Anger, rage, or violence
- Poor school performance
- Difficulty concentrating
- Learning disability
- Pallor
- Anemia
- Fatigue
- Clumsiness
- Falling
- Tingling, burning, "pins and needles," or painful sensations in the arms, legs, and/or trunk
- Dizziness
- Poor balance
- Abnormal gait

7

Inborn Errors of B_{12} Metabolism: When Gene Defects Can Turn Deadly

So far, we've talked about the most common causes of B_{12} deficiency. But there's one more culprit we need to discuss, even though it's rarer: genetic defects. As you've seen, every cell in the body needs B_{12}. Thus, when genetic or inborn defects interfere with B_{12} metabolism, the results can be catastrophic. These defects can cause severe developmental delay, mental retardation, seizures, neurological disabilities, and even death if doctors don't identify and treat them quickly.

Nine different inherited defects can cause B_{12} deficiency. Eight of these alter the ability of cells to use B_{12} or to produce the co-enzymes needed to metabolize it, while the other one affects the transport of B_{12}. Most of the time, physicians identify these genetic errors through newborn screening. However, some children have a partial defect that screening misses. Their symptoms, undetected at birth, appear later in infancy, childhood, or even early adulthood.

WHAT DOES GENETIC B_{12} DEFICIENCY LOOK LIKE?

The signs and symptoms of B_{12} deficiency due to genetic errors are the same as for a B_{12} deficiency stemming from other causes. However, children with severe or complete gene defects often decline very rapidly in their first weeks or months of life. In addition to neurological symptoms, these infants may suffer from vomiting and diarrhea. They typically are lethargic, refuse to eat, and fail to thrive. Some of them may appear to have leukemia or immune deficiency. They can quickly lapse into a coma and die if they don't get emergency treatment.

A QUICK SCIENCE LESSON

Methylmalonic acidemia is the term used to describe a group of inherited disorders of B_{12} metabolism in which the body is unable to process certain proteins and fats properly. People with this disease may have a complete or partial deficiency of the following two enzymes (*methylmalonyl-CoA mutase, methylmalonyl-CoA epimerase*), or a defect in the transport of its cofactor (*adenosylcobalamin*). Any defect will interfere with metabolizing a substance called *methylmalonic-coenzyme A* into *succinyl-CoA*. The result is a build-up of *methylmalonic acid* (MMA) in the body, damaging tissues and organs. Symptoms may present at different ages, can range from mild to severe, and can include intellectual disabilities, metabolic acidosis, coma, and death.

B_{12} (hydroxocobalamin) therapy significantly improves methylmalonyl-CoA mutase activity, and therefore is the treatment for B_{12}-responsive methylmalonic acidemia. A low-protein diet and other nutritional cofactors are also used to manage this condition. Methylmalonic acidemia is reported to occur in 1 in 25,000 to 48,000 people, but the precise incidence is not known.

Because intervention is urgent, any infants who exhibit failure to thrive or develop neurological symptoms should be tested for B_{12} deficiency and inborn errors of B_{12} metabolism, despite negative newborn screening. This includes any child on the autism spectrum. And children, teens, and young adults with neurological symptoms also need to be screened for these defects.

Such testing rarely occurs, however, because few doctors are familiar with these conditions. Says genetic pediatric researcher Piero Rinaldo, M.D., "As a matter of fact, you cannot diagnose what you don't know, and unfortunately a large proportion of cases remain undiagnosed because these disorders are not yet included in mainstream medical practice."[1] This oversight can have fatal medical consequences—and horrifying legal consequences as well.

1 P. Rinaldo, quoted in "Spotlight on Childhood Diseases," Mayo Clinic website, www.mayoclinic.com.

—

In 1989, Patricia Stallings rushed her infant son, Ryan, to the emergency department, after he became lethargic, vomited his food, and developed trouble breathing. Lab tests ordered by the hospital's doctors showed the presence of ethylene glycol (a substance found in antifreeze) in Ryan's blood. Believing that Stallings had tried to poison Ryan, the authorities placed him in foster care, allowing Patricia only brief visits, during which she could hold and feed him. Shortly after one of these visits, Ryan became desperately ill and was rushed to the hospital, where he died. Suspecting Stallings of again poisoning her son, police arrested her. A jury convicted her of first-degree murder and Patricia went to prison. At the time, she was pregnant with her second son—a child who would be the key to her freedom.

Patricia's second child, David, entered foster care immediately after his birth. Shortly afterward, he began developing symptoms eerily similar to Ryan's. David's doctors diagnosed him with methylmalonic acidemia, an inborn error of B_{12} metabolism, and immediately began appropriate treatment.

Concerned that he might have sent an innocent woman to prison, the attorney who prosecuted Patricia Stallings consulted with several doctors and finally asked Dr. Piero Rinaldo to investigate. Dr. Rinaldo conclusively determined that Ryan's symptoms, like his brother's, stemmed from methylmalonic acidemia. The two labs that analyzed Ryan's blood had used older techniques that confused one of the substances elevated in Ryan's disorder with ethylene glycol.

The prosecutor dismissed the charges against Patricia Stallings, but by then she'd lost a year of her life for the "crime" of having a baby with an inborn error of B_{12} metabolism. Worse yet, Rinaldo says, the incorrect treatment implemented by Ryan's doctors in response to the misdiagnosis of poisoning most likely contributed to his death.[2]

—

2 Ibid.

As in Patricia Stallings' case, inborn errors of B$_{12}$ metabolism can affect more than one child in a family. Clinicians should consider inborn errors of B$_{12}$ metabolism as a possibility in patients who are critically ill with unclear clinical and biochemical findings, particularly when there is a suspicious family history, or a previous sibling death. Detecting such errors early can often prevent multiple tragedies.

Because some of these inborn errors don't respond to B$_{12}$ therapy, it's critical for doctors to determine precisely which defect is present. Thus, doctors need to do sensitive genetic testing to properly diagnose children with any of these errors.

COBALAMIN C DISEASE: THE MOST COMMON B$_{12}$ GENE FLAW

An in-depth look at inborn errors of B$_{12}$ metabolism is far beyond the scope of this book.[3] However, we'd like to take a quick look at one genetic defect in particular.

Cobalamin C (cblC) disease, the most common inborn error of B$_{12}$ metabolism, is also called *methylmalonic aciduria with homocystinuria*. In this genetic defect, both methylmalonic acid and homocysteine build up in the body, causing potentially life-threatening disease.[4] It is responsive to hydroxocobalamin therapy.

Cobalamin C disease can strike at different ages, and symptoms can range from mild to severe. Most people show initial symptoms within the first year of life, but symptoms can also show up in older children, teens, or young adults. Fasting, illness, infection, or eating large amounts of protein will often trigger symptoms.

---

3 If you are a doctor or lay reader interested in learning more about the gene defects that can cause B$_{12}$ deficiency, we recommend *Disorders of Intracellular Cobalamin Metabolism*, by Nuria Carrillo-Carrasco, M.D., David Adams, M.D., Ph.D., and Charles P. Venditti, M.D., Ph.D.

4 T. Kuhne, R. Bubl, and R. Baumgartner, "Maternal Vegan Diet Causing a Serious Infantile Neurological Disorder Due to Vitamin B$_{12}$ Deficiency," *European Journal of Pediatrics* 150 (1991): 205–8.

Symptoms of Cobalamin C Disease in Newborns and Infants Can Include:

- Poor appetite and growth; vomiting
- Lethargy or excessive sleepiness
- Low muscle tone (floppy muscles and joints)
- Seizures or infantile spasms
- Microcephaly (small head and brain size)
- Intrauterine growth retardation
- Hydrocephalus ("water on the brain") and other brain abnormalities
- Megaloblastic anemia
- Developmental delays or mental retardation
- Vision, heart, and kidney problems/defects
- Nystagmus, retinopathy
- Skin rashes
- Pallor
- Neurological abnormalities
- Hemolytic uremic syndrome (HUS), a dangerous syndrome involving kidney damage and destruction of red blood cells.

In toddlers, symptoms can also include low blood cell counts, megaloblastic anemia, global delays, brain dysfunction or damage, and poor muscle tone. In adults, symptoms can include mental or behavioral problems, psychosis, progressive cognitive decline, tremor, and weakness in the arms or legs. Tests may also show degeneration of the spinal cord.

Cobalamin C disease is incurable, but early treatment with hydroxocobalamin injections, a low-protein diet, and other prescribed nutritional supplements can dramatically reduce its effects. If patients don't receive this treatment, they can be crippled for life or even die.

———

Evan was hospitalized at 6 weeks of age. He had trouble breathing, was feverish, and had anemia. A few days later, his doctors discharged him.

At age 2, Evan again arrived at the ER. At that time, he was eating poorly and failing to thrive, and his weight was under the 5th percentile. His pediatrician had diagnosed anemia and treated it with iron supplements.

The ER doctor admitted Evan to the hospital's pediatric ward for observation. Routine blood work revealed significantly elevated serum lactate dehydrogenase, an indicator of injury or disease. All other blood work was normal, and there was no anemia. A chest X-ray showed marked lung scarring and a normal heart size.

While he was in the hospital, Evan started deteriorating further. He began suffering from respiratory distress and started wheezing. An echocardiogram was abnormal, and a CAT scan of his chest revealed signs of pulmonary hypertension (high blood pressure in the arteries leading from the heart to the lungs, which is an extremely dangerous condition). Doctors transferred him to the pediatric cardiac unit and started him on medications to improve his heart and lung function.

Evan's doctors found out that his 3-year-old brother Luke had a history of hemolytic uremic syndrome (HUS), a potentially deadly disorder that can be caused by cobalamin C disease. Testing indeed showed that Evan had cobalamin C disease, and his doctors immediately started treatment.

Four days after his treatment started, Evan's blood tests markedly improved. But in the ICU, his condition worsened. He went into a pulmonary hypertensive crisis, and his heart stopped. Resuscitation efforts were unsuccessful, and Evan died.

Evan's doctors suspected that he had severe damage to the vessels in his lungs as the result of chronic high homocysteine levels caused by his cobalamin C disease. Chronic high homocysteine damages blood vessels, promoting vasoconstriction. In the lungs, this causes symptoms of wheezing and labored breathing, and leads to increased pulmonary pressures and pulmonary embolisms (blood clots that migrate to the lung).

Evan's tragic death saved his older brother, Luke. After Evan's death, doctors checked Luke and found that he had the same genetic defect. The doctors report that as a result of treatment, Luke "had almost complete normalization of metabolic abnormalities without the appearance of neurological signs at follow-up."[5]

The deadly consequences of a single oversight

How important is it for doctors to be knowledgeable about inborn errors of B12 metabolism? Evan might still be alive today if his pediatrician had looked for a B12 problem when he spotted the child's anemia and poor development. And Patricia Stallings might now have two healthy children—and would have been spared a year in jail for a crime she never committed.

Cases like this show how critical it is for children to receive in-depth screening for B12-related problems when they develop failure to thrive, developmental delay, developmental regression, seizures, or other neurological symptoms. These tests—described in detail in Chapter 11—can identify both common causes of B12 deficiency and the much rarer genetic defects that can ruin a young life . . . or even end it.

Johnny, an 8-year-old boy from Chicago, arrived at the emergency department (ED) with a history of mental status changes over a four-week period. Previously, he'd been healthy and had developed normally. Johnny's parents told the hospital staff that he first lost

5 F. G. Iodice et al., "Cobalamin C Defect Presenting with Isolated Pulmonary Hypertension," *Pediatrics* 132, no. 1 (July 2013): e248–51. DOI: 10.1542/peds.2012-1945. Epub 2013 Jun 10.

the ability to answer simple questions, and then the ability to follow commands. He also lost the ability to complete simple tasks such as brushing his teeth. His speech became hesitant, and he had difficulty pronouncing words. Finally, his spontaneous speech disappeared altogether. He also started having trouble sleeping, and slept for only two to three hours at night. Two weeks before coming to the emergency department, Johnny was evaluated by a psychiatrist and treated with Prozac.

The doctors in the ED noted that Johnny's mood fluctuated widely and he would not make eye contact. He was unable to act or make decisions, which is characteristic of certain psychotic and neurotic conditions. He had no spontaneous speech, and while he could answer some simple questions, he had trouble following simple commands. He also had spontaneous inappropriate outbursts of laughter and crying.

The doctors ordered an array of diagnostic tests, including extensive blood work, a lumbar puncture with spinal fluid analysis, an electroencephalography (EEG), and a brain MRI. Johnny's brain MRI showed mild to moderate volume loss (brain shrinkage). The EEG showed a slow rhythm and marked slow wave abnormalities over the frontal lobe.

Johnny was treated with Ativan, and briefly improved. Then he was treated with fosphenytoin (an anti-seizure drug) and became agitated, developed a fast heart rate, became more confused, and started having episodes of breath holding.

Doctors started Johnny on another anti-seizure drug to improve his sleep cycle. He was still delirious and began having difficulty sitting and walking without assistance. He was treated with a steroid, followed by intravenous immune globulin for presumed autoimmune encephalopathy (brain disease or malfunction). He was then transferred to an inpatient rehabilitation hospital, where his confusion and delirium improved slightly.

Nine days after discharge, Johnny began having visual hallucinations. Three days later, an ambulance brought him back to the emer-

gency department in status epilepticus—a life-threatening medical condition in which epileptic seizures follow one another without recovery of consciousness between them. At this point, doctors began to look for other possible causes of Johnny's mental regression, including inborn errors of B_{12} metabolism. Tests showed that his methylmalonic acid and homocysteine were both extremely elevated at 35,680 μmol/L (normal 87–318) and 109 μmol/L (normal 1.2–9.6) respectively. Further evaluation revealed that Johnny had cobalamin C disease.

The doctors started treatment including a low-protein diet, daily injections of hydroxycobalamin, and oral carnitine and betaine. Over the next five months, Johnny improved and his MMA and homocysteine levels dropped significantly. However, he continued to have episodes of disorientation and nonsensical speech. He also had difficulty walking, and was discharged to an inpatient rehabilitation facility.

A follow-up two months later showed that Johnny's psychiatric and cognitive symptoms had resolved, and his gait had improved. Johnny's brother Peter was also tested and found to have the same genetic defect. Peter had a milder case of cobalamin C disease, and his physical exam revealed a subtle spasticity.[6]

———

Early diagnosis of cobalamin C disease is critical because an effective treatment regimen exists. In 2004, many states began to include screening for methylmalonic acidemia in their newborn screening. But parents and health-care providers need to be aware that cobalamin defects (especially partial defects) can be missed on mass spectrometry screening. Test results are often based on elevated propionylcarnitine (C3) levels, and cutoff levels vary. In the case we discussed above, a retrospective review of Johnny's C3 newborn blood spot revealed a concentration of 8.49 μM/L (normal 0.0100–8.00). Peter's newborn screening C3 was 6.77 μM/L (which

6 Krueger JM, et al. A treatable metabolic cause of encephalopathy: cobalamin C deficiency in an 8-Year-Old Male. *Pediatrics*. Originally published online, December 15, 2014; DOI: 10.1542/peds.2013-1427. http://pediatrics.aappublications.org/content/early/2014/12/09/peds.2013-1427

is considered normal). Thus, errors of B$_{12}$ metabolism must *always* be considered early in the differential diagnosis of any infant, child, or teen with neurologic or psychiatric symptoms, and tests must be repeated. In these metabolic defects, serum B$_{12}$ values will be normal and methylmalonic acid testing must always be included and/or repeated, despite normal newborn screening.

It may be imprecise to classify cobalamin C disease into two phenotypes depending on age of presentation (early-onset vs. late-onset). In some late-onset cases, earlier symptoms may have gone unrecognized or may have been misdiagnosed. According to the literature, early-onset cobalamin C disease involves *in utero* changes, and symptoms appear in infants or toddlers. Late-onset cobalamin C disease is believed to occur in otherwise previously healthy older children, teens, or adults, who then develop neurologic, psychiatric, and cognitive symptoms. It is possible that the late-onset individuals have a milder form of the disease that goes undetected in their early years because their symptoms are assumed to be quirky behavior or are misdiagnosed as a psychiatric or autism spectrum disorder. These people often are diagnosed following an infection, prolonged fasting, dehydration, or stress, because even minor challenges to their systems can make them seriously ill.

Long-term management of cobalamin C disease involves reducing the metabolic derangement by lowering plasma homocysteine and methylmalonic acid concentrations and maintaining plasma methionine concentrations within the normal ranges. Treatment consists of parenteral or injectable hydroxocobalamin, oral betaine, and oral folate or folinic acid. Other therapeutic approaches include methionine, pyridoxine, and levocarnitine supplementation.

In Utero	Newborns & Infants	Older Children, Teens, Adults
• microcephaly • restricted growth • hydrocephalus • mild dysmorphic • features • congenital heart disease • dilated cardiomyopathy	• lethargy • poor feeding • vomiting • failure to thrive • hypotonia • hypothermia • neurological symptoms • seizures • infantile spasms • poor head growth • global developmental delay • encephalopathy • respiratory distress • ketoacidosis • hyperammonemia • neutropenia • thrombocytopenia • retinopathy	• developmental delay • neurological symptoms • pyschiatric symptoms • cognitive symptoms • seizures • subacute combined degeneration of the spinal cord • tubulointerstitial • nephritis • progressive renal failure • pancreatitis • movement disorders • immune impairment • optic nerve entropy • growth failure

Figure 7.1: Age of Presentation and Disease Characteristics of Methylmalonic Acidemia/Aciduria.

Treatment of cblC Disease:

- Injectable hydroxocobalamin[1]
- Betaine
- Folate or folinic acid[2]
- Methionine
- Pyridoxine
- Levocarnitine

Newborn Screening:

1. Propionylcarnitine (C3): Abnormal if C3 is elevated
2. Methionine: Abnormal if decreased.

Detection by newborn screening depends on the C3 and C3/C2 ratio cut-off values used by reference laboratories and availability of low methionine.[3]

Biochemical Testing to Identify Disorders of Intracellular Cobalamin Metabolism:

1. Urine and/or plasma organic acid analysis (which includes methylmalonic acid testing).
2. Plasma amino acid analysis.
3. Total plasma homocysteine analysis.

---

1 Cyanocobalamin is not to be used.
2 Folic acid is not to be used.
3 If the above tests are abnormal, the complementation group analysis test is used to identify the specific defect of intracellular cobalamin metabolism (cblA, cblB, cblC, cblD, cblE, cblF, cblG, and cblJ).

8

Lost Children: The Autism-B₁₂ Connection

Currently, the United States—along with much of the rest of the world—is in the grip of an autism epidemic. The Centers for Disease Control and Prevention recently released new figures showing that autism now affects an astonishing 1 in 68 children in the United States.[1] Other countries around the world, from Israel to Denmark, are reporting surges in autism rates as well.[2,3]

How does autism relate to B_{12} deficiency? To understand the connection, you need to know that autism isn't a specific disorder, like Down syndrome. Instead, it's a cluster of symptoms, with a variety of causes. The classic symptoms of autism include poor language acquisition or loss of language, an inability to relate to other people normally, and repetitive movements or mannerisms called *self-stimulatory behaviors* (or *stims*). Because these symptoms can be mild or severe, and individuals with autism range from severely delayed and nonverbal people to brilliant doctors and college professors, experts tend to speak of autism as a *spectrum* disorder.

Autism has a variety of causes, some known and some still a mystery. In many cases, autistic symptoms stem from gene defects, such as Fragile X syndrome or Rett syndrome. Infections before birth or during early infancy can be culprits as well. Some drugs, such as the antiseizure drug sodium valproate (Depakote),[4] can cause autism

1 www.cdc.gov/features/dsautismdata
2 www.ncbi.nlm.nih.gov/pubmed/24554161
3 www.ncbi.nlm.nih.gov/pubmed/22836322
4 Valproic acid (Depakote) is a drug commonly prescribed for seizures and mental illness. Interestingly, it is known to disturb folate and B_{12} metabolism. Thus, it should come as no surprise that valproic acid can cause functional B_{12} deficiency, giving rise to developmental delay and other intellectual disabilities that clinicians mistakenly call autism.

in children exposed *in utero*.[5,6] In addition, there's some evidence pointing to environmental toxins as a factor. Millions of cases are *idiopathic*, meaning that doctors don't know what went wrong.

But there's one culprit that's been known for decades—and yet doctors almost never spot it. If you examine the cases we describe in this book, you'll see that *every symptom of autism can stem from low B$_{12}$*. In fact, many children and adults are walking around with a label of "autism" when in reality they aren't autistic, but at some point in their development (usually in infancy), sustained a brain injury caused by vitamin B$_{12}$ deficiency. A more accurate medical term to describe these individuals is *B$_{12}$-deficiency Acquired Brain Injury (BABI)*.[7]

WHAT IS BABI?

B   B$_{12}$-deficiency

A   Acquired

B   Brain

I   Injury

An injury to the brain and/or nervous system caused by vitamin B$_{12}$ deficiency during a child's growth and development, resulting in long-term intellectual, social, and/or motor disabilities. These disabilities fall on a spectrum from mild to severe.

---

5 J. Christensen et al., "Prenatal Valproate Exposure and Risk of Autism Spectrum Disorders and Childhood Autism," *Journal of the American Medical Association* 309, no. 16 (April 2013): 1696–703. DOI: 10.1001/jama.2013.2270.

6 P. M. Haddad et al., "A Review of Valproate in Psychiatric Practice," *Expert Opinion on Drug Metabolism & Toxicology* 5, no. 5 (May 2009): 539–51. DOI: 10.1517/17425250902911455.

7 It is well documented that B$_{12}$ deficiency causes injury and abnormalities in the developing human brain is well documented, as revealed in these pages and medical literature in general. However, as of this writing, there is no official, standardized term for this problem. Accordingly, for the sake of clarity and convenience, we use the term "B$_{12}$-deficiency Acquired Brain Injury," or BABI, in describing and discussing the constellation of signs and symptoms that so closely mimic (and can easily be mistaken for) ASD. It should be understood that the term BABI is (at present) a nonstandard abbreviation employed by the authors as a service to readers for comparison's sake with ASD. Also, since BABI is considered a nonstandard term at this time, it won't necessarily be familiar to your doctor or health-care practitioners in general.

The symptoms of autism are *virtually identical* to the symptoms that stem from neurological damage due to B_{12} deficiency. Figure 8.1 shows these symptoms side by side:

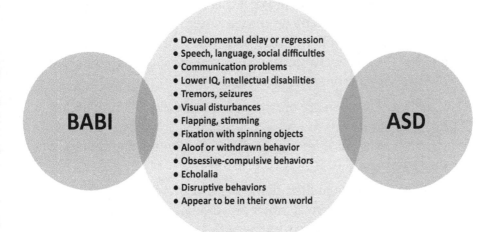

Figure 8.1. BABI vs. Autism Spectrum Disorders (ASD).

There's no way to know how many cases of autism are really BABI because doctors almost never check the serum B_{12} levels of children who develop autistic symptoms, nor do they perform more sensitive tests to rule out a deficiency or a genetic defect affecting B_{12} metabolism. Our belief, however, is that the number of cases of BABI being mistaken for autism is large and growing. Consider these facts:

- 18 percent of the U.S. population between the ages of 20 and 59 have low B_{12} or a deficiency, a number that includes many pregnant or nursing mothers.[8]

8 L. H. Allen, "How Common Is Vitamin B-12 Deficiency?" *American Journal of Clinical Nutrition* 89, no. 2 (2009): 693S–696S.

- A growing number of women in their childbearing years are adhering to B_{12}-deficient diets that drastically reduce or eliminate animal products, and many of these women are supplementing their diets incorrectly. One European study found that B_{12} deficiency among pregnant vegetarians ranged from 17 percent to 39 percent depending on the trimester.[9] Another study by the same research group, this time using the more sensitive MMA and holo-transcobalamin II tests, revealed a B_{12} deficiency rate of 62 percent among pregnant vegetarians.[10]

- Many more women are breastfeeding these days than in earlier decades. While this is a very healthful trend, babies of B_{12}-deficient mothers are at far higher risk of developing B_{12} deficiency than they would be if they received formula.

- Millions of women in their childbearing years are now taking gastric acid blocking medications, medications for diabetes, or other drugs that interfere with the body's ability to metabolize B_{12}. Additionally, more and more *children* are taking these medications.

- Increasing numbers of women are undergoing bariatric surgery for weight loss, which removes a part of the digestive system needed to process B_{12}, and many of these women are not receiving the proper high-dose, lifelong B_{12} supplementation they need following this surgery.

- Increasing numbers of women are undergoing cosmetic, dental, and other medical procedures involving nitrous oxide, which inactivates B_{12}.

- Doctors now prescribe high-dose folic acid for women before and during pregnancy, as well as during breastfeeding. Again, this is a good idea—but extra folic acid masks the signs of anemia

9 R. Pawlak et al., "How Prevalent Is Vitamin B(12) Deficiency among Vegetarians?" *Nutrition Review* 71, no. 2 (February 2013): 110–17. DOI: 10.1111/nure.12001. Epub 2013 Jan 2.
10 R. Pawlak, S. E. Lester, and T. Babatunde, "The Prevalence of Cobalamin Deficiency among Vegetarians Assessed by Serum Vitamin B₁₂: A Review of Literature," *European Journal of Clinical Nutrition* (2014): 1–8.

and macrocytosis which, while not always present in B_{12} deficiency, can alert doctors to a B_{12} problem.

- B_{12} deficiency can stem from anorexia or bulimia, which affect growing numbers of women. Women who recover from eating disorders may remain deficient in B_{12} for months or years afterward.

Collectively, these facts and statistics tell us that the number of women of childbearing age who are at risk for B_{12} deficiency has increased dramatically over the past few decades. Thus, we believe it's a certainty that the subgroup of "autistic" children who really have BABI is increasing as well. And we believe that these numbers will continue to rise until doctors begin to address this disorder and test for B_{12} deficiency whenever they suspect autism.

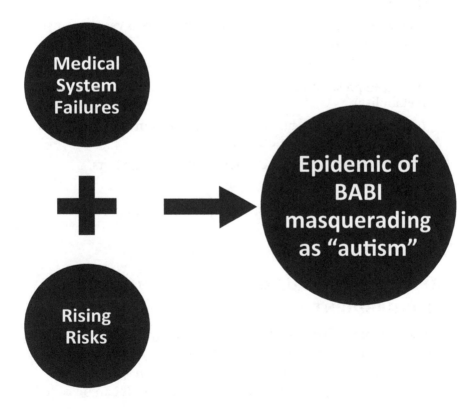

Figure 8.2. The roots of the BABI epidemic.

Medical System Failures:

1. Lack of knowledge about B_{12} deficiency.
2. Failure to screen at-risk populations.
3. Failure to screen symptomatic patients.
4. Failure to identify and properly address *MTHFR* gene mutations (see Chapter 3 for details).
5. Inadequate treatment protocols.
6. Insufficient DRI (dietary reference intakes) for B_{12} in prenatal vitamins.
7. Current laboratory threshold considered "normal" for serum B_{12} level is dangerously low.
8. Failure to use urinary MMA test to assist in diagnosis.

Rising Risks:

1. Increases in veganism/vegetarianism/lacto-ovo vegetarianism and macrobiotic diets.
2. Increase in breastfeeding.
3. Increased prescribing of drugs that impair B_{12} uptake or metabolism.
4. Increases in medical and dental procedures involving N_2O in infants, children, and mothers.
5. Higher rates of N_2O abuse in teens and young adults.
6. Higher rates of eating disorders.
7. Increase in junk food diets, poor nutrition, and processed foods.
8. Growing number of environmental toxins.

THE ALPHABET SOUP OF AUTISM IS MISSING A KEY INGREDIENT

Autism is sometimes called *childhood disintegrative disorder* (CDD) when it's diagnosed after age 3. It can go by the name of *pervasive developmental disorder* (PDD) or *autism spectrum disorder* (ASD) when symptoms are mild or atypical. It can be called

Asperger syndrome (AS) when individuals have higher IQs and fewer social impairments. If symptoms are very mild, it may be classified as *nonverbal learning disability* (NLD) or an attention problem such as *attention deficit disorder* or *attention deficit hyperactivity disorder* (ADD or ADHD).

So what's missing in this alphabet soup? The *B* for B_{12}—because any of these diagnoses may actually be B_{12} deficiency. The neurological symptoms of B_{12} deficiency can take very different forms in different children, leading to a wide variety of labels. But labels aren't treatment—and children with low B_{12} or B_{12} deficiency need treatment fast, because at some point the damage done by their deficiency will be partially or completely irreversible. Here's an example.

———

Recently, doctors published a case study about a child diagnosed with childhood disintegrative disorder (CDD). The boy, a vegetarian from a middle-class family, seemed normal until he reached 6½ years of age. One evening, he told his family he'd seen a ghost. In the days that followed, he started seeing bright flashes of lights. He became restless, distractible, irritable, and demanding.

Gradually, the boy began speaking less and less to his family. He started repeating other people's words (an autistic symptom called echolalia). As time went on, he retreated more and more into his own world. By the time he was 9, he'd stopped speaking in complete sentences. He avoided making eye contact with people and he started exhibiting "stims" like finger tapping.

The case study's authors first saw the boy when he was 14. They reported: "He appeared to be unmindful of the presence of other people, approaching them only to sniff at them or to tap the round buttons of their coats." A psychological exam showed that he was functioning socially at a 4½-year-old level and had severe mental retardation.

Lab tests revealed that the boy had a very severe B_{12} deficiency. The doctors started him on B_{12} injections, and his eye contact and pacing *behavior soon improved. Over time, his other behavioral problems grew less severe as well. The doctors conclude: "The degree of improvement shown by this child with vitamin B$_{12}$ supplementation has been quite remarkable and encouraging." However, they say that considering the length of time that elapsed between the start of his symptoms and his diagnosis, "It would be too optimistic to expect complete recovery."*[11]

Child Injured—BABI, not ASD.

—

As this case shows, BABI and ASD share many symptoms because they are both developmental brain disorders. But *BABI can be prevented if doctors perform early screening of both mom and child.* Early recognition and diagnosis of those already afflicted will result in improved neurological and cognitive outcomes. Sometimes the symptoms caused by a beginning B$_{12}$ deficiency can be completely reversed, but only if promptly diagnosed and treated. Labeling children with PDD, CDD, NLD,

> There is no valid reason for doctors to miss the symptoms of low B$_{12}$.

or any other type of autism spectrum disorder when they actually have B$_{12}$ deficiency is condemning them unnecessarily to a lifetime of disability, which is what the child presented in the above case study will most likely suffer.

This is why we strongly urge physicians and all members of the health-care team who diagnose or treat autistic and other developmentally delayed children to add two more acronyms to their diagnostic "alphabet soup." The first, as already mentioned, is BABI, or B$_{12}$-deficiency Acquired Brain Injury. And the second is ABC—which stands for the *Autism-B$_{12}$ Connection.*

11 S. Malhotra et al., "Brief Report: Childhood Disintegrative Disorder as a Likely Manifestation of Vitamin B$_{12}$ Deficiency," *Journal of Autism and Developmental Disorders* 43, no. 9 (September 2013): 2207–10. DOI: 10.1007/s10803-013-1762-6.

A HALF CENTURY OF MEDICAL LITERATURE
IGNORED

There is no valid reason for doctors to miss the symptoms of low B$_{12}$ or a diagnosis of B$_{12}$ deficiency. The medical literature over the past 50 years is filled with reports of children developing autistic-like symptoms as a result of B$_{12}$ deficiency. Here's a small sampling of recent published cases:

- In 2001, doctors diagnosed B$_{12}$ deficiency in a 15-month-old whose signs and symptoms included failure to thrive and developmental delay. Blood tests proved B$_{12}$ deficiency (low serum B$_{12}$ and elevated methylmalonic acid). At the time of the girl's diagnosis, a brain MRI revealed "global cerebral atrophy." Doctors began B$_{12}$ treatment immediately, but it was too late to undo all of the damage. At 28 months of age, her fine motor skills were at the 9-month level and her gross motor skills were comparable to those of an 18-month-old child. Her expressive language was at the 10-month level, and her receptive language was at the 12-month level. At 32 months, she'd made developmental progress but continued to have developmental delays, especially in speech and language.[12]
  Child Injured—BABI, not ASD.

- A 2014 study in the *Journal of Child Neurology* reported on 14 infants and children in whom B$_{12}$ deficiency led to developmental delay or regression. The authors report that in 57 percent of the cases, "severe to profound delay" occurred. All of the children were exclusively or primarily breastfed, and 10 of the 12 mothers proved to be low in B$_{12}$. Most of the children showed remarkable improvement after receiving treatment but did not achieve normal development.[13]
  Child Injured—BABI, not ASD.

12 R. Muhammad et al., "Neurologic Impairment in Children Associated with Maternal Dietary Deficiency of Cobalamin—Georgia, 2001," *Morbidity and Mortality Weekly Report* 52, no. 4 (January 31, 2003): 61–64).
13 R. Jain R et al., "Vitamin B$_{12}$ Deficiency in Children: A Treatable Cause of Neurodevelopmental Delay," *Journal of Child Neurology* (January 21, 2014).

85

- Another 2014 case, reported in *Paediatrics and Child Health*, involved a 7-month-old boy who stopped eating, lost weight, slept all the time, missed developmental milestones, and stopped smiling and interacting with other people. Luckily for this little boy, his alert doctors quickly tested him for B$_{12}$ deficiency and found that his B$_{12}$ level was incredibly low. It turned out that he had pernicious anemia. The doctors started treatment right away and report: "He became increasingly interactive, observant, and began to smile." He was still delayed when doctors followed up at 11 months, but at 19 months he was meeting all of his milestones.[14]
  Continue monitoring for learning and/or intellectual disabilities.

Sadly, many of the worst cases of B$_{12}$ deficiency resulting in autistic behavior or developmental delay never reach the medical literature. Here is a typical case reported by a mom who contacted us for help. (Note: This mother settled with her child's doctor out of court and has been threatened with retribution if she tells her story openly. We greatly appreciate her courage in letting us tell her story.)

———

Jason was born in the mid-1990s after a normal pregnancy. Before his mother (a teacher) became pregnant, she asked her doctor to check her iron level because she knew she tended to be anemic, but her doctor said her test results were normal.

Jason was a happy, healthy-looking baby. He met all his milestones and was smiling and alert by 12 weeks of age. He developed normally over the first six months and responded eagerly to the people around him. The only symptoms his mom noticed were mouth ulcers, which cleared up quickly, and frequent infections.

14 K. McNeil K et al., "Vitamin B$_{12}$ Deficiency with Intrinsic Factor Antibodies in an Infant with Poor Growth and Developmental Delay," *Paediatric & Child Health* 19, no. 2 (February 2014): 84–86.

After the 6-month mark, things began to change. At Jason's checkup, the doctor noted that his length and head circumference had dropped to the 5th percentile. The doctor noticed another unusual sign: Jason failed to turn his head toward sounds.

Around that time, Jason started vomiting up large amounts of breast milk. But he wouldn't take a bottle, so breastfeeding was his mom's only option. He was also becoming lethargic, sleeping up to 17 hours a day. When he was awake, he had no energy and didn't want to play with his toys.

Worried about these changes in her once bright and happy child, Jason's mom made an appointment with a pediatrician. At her appointment, she brought up the question of anemia, but the doctor said that babies do not suffer from anemia even if their mothers are anemic. She asked the doctor to do blood tests, but he replied that he didn't like to do tests on babies because the tests didn't do any good and only caused the babies pain. He made a referral to a speech therapist because of Jason's delayed language, but he concluded that "time would be kind" and solve Jason's problems.

But time wasn't kind. Instead, Jason grew sicker and sicker. He started making a low crying sound when he was awake. He stopped looking at people's faces and instead focused on lights. He wouldn't hold a rattle or reach for his toys. And when his mom sat him up, he slumped to one side.

Desperate, Jason's mom took him to another doctor who suggested that he wasn't ill but intellectually delayed. Then she took him back to the pediatrician, who repeated that he didn't want to do "nasty" tests that would hurt Jason.

Reluctantly, the pediatrician admitted Jason to the hospital, where blood tests were done. Explaining the test results, the pediatrician commented that Jason didn't have small red blood cells (a sign of iron-deficiency anemia) but instead had enlarged cells. Apparently, the doctor thought these enlarged blood cells were a normal sign, when in fact they are a common sign of B_{12} deficiency. Jason was discharged from the hospital, even though an MRI showed abnormalities in his brain and he was still very ill.

Jason's mom finally took him to another city to see a pediatric neurologist. This doctor, too, initially believed that Jason had a developmental disability. However, when he saw the difference between Jason's current state and photos his mom provided of Jason as an alert, happy young infant, he agreed to admit Jason to a hospital.

At the new hospital, doctors ordered blood tests. Within four hours after the tests were completed, a hematologist (a doctor who specializes in blood disorders) showed up in Jason's room with a diagnosis: life-threatening B₁₂ deficiency, requiring immediate treatment. Further testing confirmed that Jason had a severe deficiency, and later tests showed that his mother had pernicious anemia.

Jason received aggressive treatment for his B₁₂ deficiency. His health improved, but it was too late to repair all of the damage to his brain. At age 5, he had the language skills of a 2½-year-old and an IQ of 46. By the age of 9, he received a diagnosis of autism.

Now that Jason is 20, his mother worries that he won't be able to hold a job. "He just can't commit to turning up to work every day," she says. "He is unreliable and unpredictable. He is often confused about what he wants to do, and although he has a lovely girlfriend, he doesn't have the necessary social skills that are needed to treat her as a normal boyfriend would treat his girlfriend."

She adds, "When people meet Jason they don't know or see that anything is not normal immediately. He is a good-looking young man who enjoys bike riding and other physical activities. But, as soon as a conversation is initiated, it is obvious he thinks at a different level than the average 20-year-old. He still calls me 'mummy' and he takes my hand and directs me to scratch his back or run my fingers through his hair. He is very obsessive with how things need to be done, and when."

Jason has many autistic rituals and odd behaviors. For instance, his family has to hide their car keys because he loves to watch them start the car with jumper cables. So if he gets his hands on their keys, he sneaks into the car and turns on the lights to run down the battery.

Jason's mom concludes, "We love him dearly, and we are well aware that we are lucky that he did manage to get through what was potentially a life-threatening situation. But it breaks my heart to know that all of this could have been prevented . . . if only."

Child Injured—BABI, not ASD.

———

Often, even if a true diagnosis of B_{12} deficiency is finally made, children are still mislabeled as "autistic" and placed in classrooms for children with autism, and physicians may even code these cases incorrectly under autism spectrum disorders. Many teachers and therapists working with "autistic" children have no idea that some of their students are not autistic, but actually have "autistic-like" behaviors, mannerisms, or developmental delays caused by a B_{12}-deficiency acquired brain injury (BABI). Frequently, parents are not even told by their children's physicians that chronic untreated B_{12} deficiency is what caused their children's disability, and that these children are not autistic, though they certainly share similar social impairments and learning disabilities.

This problem may be occurring because doctors fear that medical services or therapies will not be paid, or that autism programs will exclude such B_{12}-deficient children from needed services. It also may be due to fear of a malpractice lawsuit. And some doctors may mistakenly believe that a child has concurrent B_{12} deficiency and autism, failing to understand how true B_{12} deficiency gives rise to intellectual disabilities and therefore causes autistic-like behaviors.

Of course, any child who has a developmental delay or an intellectual disability stemming from any cause (for instance, traumatic brain injury, Down syndrome, Fragile X syndrome, stroke, or autism) will benefit from receiving a variety of therapies to improve lost function, and this applies to BABI children as well. But categorizing children with BABI as autistic merely helps to hide the epidemic of B_{12} deficiency, sentencing additional children and future generations to permanent disability.

Another problem may be that the medical community doesn't realize that some BABI children are actually a subset of patients with subacute combined degeneration, or SCD (see Chapter 6 for information on this condition). SCD is often diagnosed late in adults, and children are even less likely to receive an accurate diagnosis—especially when doctors already have the convenient classification of "autism."

DOCTORS SEE ONLY PART OF THE PICTURE

So far, we've looked at cases in which doctors have completely missed diagnoses of B$_{12}$ deficiency. However, there are other cases in which doctors identify a B$_{12}$ deficiency in children with "autism" but still fail to see the full picture.

For instance, consider a recent case report in *Pediatrics*. In it, doctors describe three children with autism who also suffered a gradual loss of vision, going from apparently normal vision to near blindness. The clinicians who wrote up their case studies discovered that all three children had B$_{12}$ deficiency and provided quick treatment, resulting in a restoration of normal vision. Their conclusion: The children's restricted diets led to their B$_{12}$ deficiency.[15]

In our opinion, that's very short-sighted. Why? Because it's a virtual certainty that these children's "autistic" symptoms, and not just their later vision problems, stemmed from B$_{12}$ deficiency. In patients with B$_{12}$ deficiency, behavioral and developmental problems often emerge many months or years earlier than visual symptoms. Most likely, all three of these children were deficient from infancy or early childhood and their undiagnosed and untreated deficiency worsened over time. Eating a poor diet didn't help the matter, but eating table foods with adequate B$_{12}$ simply would not have been enough to correct the underlying deficiency. Aggressive B$_{12}$ replacement therapy was required.

15 S. L. Pineles, R. A. Avery, and G. T. Liu, "Vitamin B$_{12}$ Optic Neuropathy in Autism," *Pediatrics* 126, no. 4 (October 2010): e967–70. DOI: 10.1542/peds.2009-2975. Epub 2010 Sep 20.

ONE MORE FACTOR IN THE AUTISM-B$_{12}$ CONNECTION: *MTHFR*

In Chapter 3, we talked about the *MTHFR* gene. Common mutations in this gene can put a person at much higher risk for B$_{12}$ deficiency.

A recent study found that children with autism were much more likely to have defective copies of the *MTHFR* gene than other children. The researchers reported that 25 percent of children with ASD had a combination of two mutated genes (C677T and A1298C), compared to only 15 percent of controls. Having both of these mutations is thought to lower the MTHFR enzyme's activity by about 50 to 60 percent. The researchers also found that 98 percent of children with ASD had at least one abnormal *MTHFR* gene.[16] The researchers say that while defective *MTHFR* genes in and of themselves are unlikely to account for the majority of autism risk, rising rates of autism may stem in part from environmental factors that expose this genetic vulnerability.

From our point of view, more research needs to be done on *MTHFR* mutations in the general public as well as the autism population. Children with defective *MTHFR* genes may be more vulnerable to BABI. This is especially true if they have other risk factors (for instance, a vegetarian diet or N$_2$O exposure), or if their mothers were B$_{12}$-deficient during pregnancy and/or breastfeeding. Remember, there are many people who have *MTHFR* mutations and do not have autism, as well as many people who have BABI and do not have these mutations. Therefore, *MTHFR* mutations are only *one* of many established risk factors contributing to BABI. However, it could be that this mutation is another variable that makes some children more vulnerable to BABI, especially if they have other risk factors.

---

16 M. Boris et al., "Association of *MTHFR* Gene Variants with Autism," *Journal of American Physicians and Surgeons* 9, no. 4 (winter 2004): 106–8.

THE UNKNOWN TOLL OF BABI

How many children with BABI are being condemned to a life-long misdiagnosis of autism? We will never know the answer to this question unless we look for it. Currently, most medical professionals are unaware of the neuropsychiatric manifestations of B_{12} deficiency and the role that this deficiency plays in developmental disorders—and, in particular, the symptoms labeled as "autism."

Stunningly, many doctors don't even know that children *can* be B_{12} deficient. In Jason's case, above, his doctor claimed that "babies do not suffer from anemia." In a similar case we describe in depth in Chapter 14, a child named Lennon became "autistic" after doctors failed to detect his B_{12} deficiency. Lennon's mother remembers bringing up B_{12} deficiency to her pediatrician on three different occasions because she had read about it in the *American Medical Association Family Medical Guide*. Her pediatrician repeatedly dismissed her input and reassured her, "Nobody gets a B_{12} deficiency. He is getting enough from your milk." He wasn't, and he nearly died. Today, he is diagnosed as autistic and needs therapy to master the simple tasks that most children his age can do easily.

A small minority of doctors, however, *are* aware that there is a link between B_{12} deficiency and autism. Unfortunately, these doctors typically prescribe high-dose vitamin B_{12} to autistic children without first performing tests to determine these children's B_{12} status. These doctors, while well intentioned, are actually preventing us from obtaining crucial information about the role B_{12} deficiency plays in autism. In addition, they are perpetuating the inaccurate diagnosis of autism in cases of BABI, because treating a child without first doing proper testing makes it impossible to document a deficiency. The same is true of parents who treat children on the autism spectrum with B_{12} without first having these children tested. *Both parents and doctors must refrain from giving a therapeutic trial or introducing B_{12} before testing.*

In addition, both doctors and parents should refrain from starting other interventions at the same time that B_{12} treatment is initiated. Starting multiple treatments at the same time can make it appear as if other therapies are helping when improvements may be due solely to the B_{12} treatments. This can lead parents to continue expensive and unnecessary treatments such as chelation or hyperbaric oxygen therapy.

A NOTE ABOUT TESTING

In some cases, young children who have low B_{12} or a B_{12} deficiency during development may at some point begin to get small amounts of B_{12} from formula or table foods, or higher doses from supplements given by parents or clinicians. As a result, they may have normal lab results. This is because there was a failure to detect and document low B_{12} or a deficiency when it occurred. This can happen for the following reasons:

- A mother who was low in B_{12} during early pregnancy or throughout pregnancy began bottle feeding.
- A mother whose breast milk was low in B_{12} stopped breastfeeding.
- A child became deficient due to exposure to nitrous oxide but over time received enough B_{12} to correct his or her deficit.
- A vegan or vegetarian mom began giving her child foods with B_{12}.
- A mother started giving her child a multivitamin, B vitamins, or high-dose B_{12} as a trial, without getting the child tested.
- A doctor prescribed multivitamins or oral B_{12} to a child without first testing the child.
- A doctor gave injectable B_{12} as a trial without first testing the child.

Remember that before *any* B_{12} is given as a trial for autistic symptoms or developmental delay, sensitive urine methylmalonic acid testing *must always* be performed.

Because the medical community ignores the problem of B$_{12}$ deficiency or at best offers hit-or-miss treatments to at-risk children without testing them, hundreds of thousands of B$_{12}$-deficient children are going undiagnosed, misdiagnosed, or undertreated. It is crucial that we begin to investigate the true incidence of B$_{12}$ deficiency in children—particularly those with symptoms of autism or developmental disability—and in women of childbearing age, so we can determine the magnitude of the problem and take steps to address it. In the 21st century, there is no excuse for allowing a child to develop BABI or "autism" as a result of a vitamin deficiency that can be prevented and successfully treated if identified early.

9

Breakdown: B_{12} Deficiency and Mental Illness

Every thought you have, and every emotion you feel, is the miraculous result of a delicate dance of neurochemicals in your brain. But a B_{12} deficiency can turn that perfect waltz of brain chemicals into chaos, leading to fuzzy thinking, irrational behavior, or even outright mental illness. As a result, you or your child may receive a diagnosis of depression, paranoia, attention deficit disorder, obsessive-compulsive disorder, or even autism or schizophrenia.

While B_{12} deficiency may not cause most cases of mental illness, it plays a powerful role in many, particularly in those involving depression or bipolar disorder. We don't know the true incidence because children and adults

> Low levels of B_{12} can cause severe mental symptoms.

aren't being screened for B_{12} deficiency when symptoms of mental illness develop—a dangerous and costly oversight.

Pediatricians, psychiatrists, and psychologists tend to use diagnostic terms to describe children with abnormal behavior or mental illness that differ from those they might apply to adults. For instance, a child who is fidgety and hyperactive may be given a diagnosis of attention deficit disorder (ADD) or attention deficit hyperactivity disorder (ADHD), whereas an adult with the same symptoms may receive a diagnosis of anxiety. A child who appears apathetic or depressed, or cannot concentrate or communicate well, may be diagnosed with a learning disability while an adult with similar signs and symptoms might be diagnosed with depression. Bear this in mind while reading this chapter.

It would be odd to see a 6-year-old given the diagnosis of depression or bipolar disorder, even though they may appear depressed or manic. But if a psychiatrist or pediatrician does diagnose your child with *any* psychiatric disorder—a medical reason, such as vitamin B$_{12}$ deficiency, merits serious consideration.

———

Ricky, a playful 7-year-old, began exhibiting changes in behavior over several months. He developed obsessive-compulsive behaviors that included repetitive stair climbing and lining up objects.

Eventually, Ricky began to fall behind in school and started having difficulty concentrating. Over time, he developed an abnormal gait, which led to a referral to a neurologist. Ricky proved to have a severe B$_{12}$ deficiency—not obsessive-compulsive disorder, depression, or attention deficit disorder.[1]

———

Brian, a once-energetic 10-year-old, was taken to the emergency department by his parents when he developed progressive difficulty in walking. He had no history of trauma, fever, or other signs of illness. A neurological evaluation showed that Brian's mental status and mood were abnormal and he had a wide-based and wobbly gait. He had to look at the position of his feet when he walked and was unable to walk in the dark, suggesting involvement of the spinal cord (common in advanced B$_{12}$ deficiency).

Brian indeed proved to have severe B$_{12}$ deficiency. Two weeks after treatment, his mental status and mood improved. One month later, he could walk normally.[2]

1 J. R. Crawford and D. Say, "Vitamin B$_{12}$ Deficiency Presenting as Acute Ataxia," *British Medical Journal Case Reports* (2013). DOI: 10.1136/bcr-2013-008840.
2 L. J. Wolansky et al., "Subacute Combined Degeneration of the Spinal Cord: MRI Detection of Preferential Involvement of the Posterior Columns in a Child," *Pediatric Radiology* 25 (1995): 140–41.

———

In Chapter 8, we briefly discussed a child who was misdiagnosed with a form of autism called CDD. The child (Matthew) began developing mental symptoms at age 6. He was fearful of ghosts, unable to sleep, and became increasingly restless. Months later he became increasingly disruptive at school, which he by then attended irregularly. His continued outbursts resulted in him not attending school at all. But even at home, he was easily distractible, irritable, demanding, and unable to sit still.

Matthew's doctor placed him on Prozac and Haldol. A year later, Matthew appeared to be in his own world, interacting only with his family. By the age of 8, he spent most his time pacing around and talking to himself. By the age of 9, he gradually stopped speaking in complete sentences. Six months later, he began making stereotypical movements such as finger tapping. Matthew was taken to additional physicians and psychiatrists, but without any benefit.

What was wrong with Matthew? Was he mentally ill, psychotic, demented, or autistic? No, just an innocent child injured on the watch of an ignorant medical system. Matthew at age 14 was diagnosed with a severe B_{12} deficiency. His serum B_{12} was only 102 pg/mL. Psychological testing found Matthew to be functioning at a 4-year-old level.

Treatment did improve Matthew's pacing, touching, and tapping to a great extent, and his echolalia and repetitive activities diminished. However his social skills, speech, and other mental abilities remained seriously delayed.[3]

———

3 S. Malhotra et al., "Brief Report: Childhood Disintegrative Disorder as a Likely Manifestation of Vitamin B_{12} Deficiency," *Journal of Autism and Developmental Disorders* 43, no. 9 (September 2013): 2207–10. DOI: 10.1007/s10803-013-1762-6.

WHY B$_{12}$ DEFICIENCY CAN CAUSE MENTAL ILLNESS

Clearly, low levels of B$_{12}$ can cause severe mental symptoms. To help you understand why, here's a quick lesson in physiology. The neurons in your brain communicate using chemicals called *neurotransmitters* to send signals from cell to cell. These chemicals include serotonin, dopamine, epinephrine, and norepinephrine, among others.

Here's how the process works. When stimulated, a sending neuron releases neurotransmitters, which enter a space called a *synapse* between the sending and receiving neurons. These neurotransmitters then bind to receptors on the receiving neuron and trigger a response. The nature of a given response depends on the neurotransmitter involved and the specific function of the receptor type it binds to.

Once a neurotransmitter does its job, the sending neuron reabsorbs it in a process called *reuptake*. This allows the sending cell to reuse its chemical messengers. Some medications, called *reuptake inhibitors*, work by decreasing this reabsorption, thereby increasing the amount of neurotransmitters remaining in the synaptic space.

If you don't have enough neurotransmitters in your brain, your neurons won't be able to communicate efficiently, and certain deficiencies are going to affect your mood, thinking, and behavior. In particular, low levels of serotonin and norepinephrine in the synapse are associated with depression and sadness. While drugs may increase the availability of these chemicals in the synapse, there still won't be enough if your body can't make them initially.

This is where B$_{12}$ comes in. Without enough B$_{12}$, your body can't synthesize all the neurotransmitters it needs. B$_{12}$ works hand in hand with several amino acids in the metabolic pathways for serotonin, dopamine, epinephrine, and norepinephrine synthesis, and low B$_{12}$ can lead to reduced levels of any or all of these crucial chemicals. That's why mental or psychological symptoms are one of the most common results of low B$_{12}$ or B$_{12}$ deficiency.

But that's not the whole story. In addition, B_{12} plays a key role in the production of antioxidants that protect your cells (including your brain cells) from toxins and destructive byproducts of metabolism, allowing these cells to stay healthy and function normally. As we noted in Chapter 3, it's also a building block of s-adenosylmethionine (SAMe), a substance that's often low in people with depression. And as we've explained, your body needs adequate B_{12} to produce the myelin insulation surrounding your neurons. Otherwise, like frayed electrical wires, these neurons can't transmit messages correctly.

For all of these reasons and more, B_{12} deficiency can make you feel and act "crazy." Sadly, when B_{12}-deficient patients develop psychiatric symptoms, doctors typically don't consider the possibility that low B_{12} might be the cause. Instead, they generally go no further than applying labels such as depression, anxiety, dementia, or obsessive-compulsive disorder and prescribing expensive drugs. One telling fact is that the majority of patients we identify with vitamin B_{12} deficiency in our own emergency departments are on antidepressants, antianxiety medications, or mood stabilizers. This reveals that their primary care doctors and other specialists failed to screen for B_{12} deficiency as a reason for their psychiatric symptoms—or were aware of a deficiency, but simply chose to disregard it.

In fact, physicians frequently fail to think of B_{12} deficiency when they examine mentally ill patients, even when other devastating signs of low B_{12} are present. In doing so, they allow a deficiency to continue damaging brain cells and altering levels of brain chemicals. As a result, their patients can suffer terribly for months or even years, as the next case shows.

—

One woman who shared her story with us is Angie, whose saga began with a lap-band operation in 2001 when she was 24 years old. This operation can lead to severe B_{12} deficiency if patients don't receive lifelong supplementation after their surgery. Unfortunately, Angie's surgeon and other doctors didn't tell her this and failed to monitor her properly.

In 2006, Angie met her future husband, Mark. She became pregnant, but suffered a miscarriage after just a few weeks. A year later, Angie started having serious memory problems and anxiety. She also lost another baby. "I was constantly dizzy and tired," she says. "I ended up passing out a few times in the same week at work. I was put on paid leave by my boss and sent home to get this figured out." But the doctors couldn't find anything wrong with her.

"I was having an increasingly difficult time focusing on work," she says. "I felt like everyone was out to get me. The headaches, the dizzy spells, being tired all the time—and then pregnancy number three failed." Fortunately, Mark stood by her. "I got married in January 2009 to the most supportive man I have ever met," she says.

At that point, Angie went back to school and earned a paralegal degree, juggling school and a job. Tragically, however, she lost two more babies in 2009. "I had no energy at this time," she says. "I was so depressed and feeling lost with my life."

Angie began suffering from muscle cramps. "I felt like a walking charley horse," as she described it. Her hands were cold all the time. She was passing out, and she began losing bladder control. In 2010, she became pregnant one more time and almost made it to 19 weeks. But one morning when she got up to walk the dog, she wound up passing out and falling down the stairs. She lost the baby and has a large scar on her face that she says "will remind me of that day for the rest of my life."

Angie's doctors said she was depressed and tried to put her on Prozac, Zoloft, and Abilify. She refused to take the medications "because I knew I was not depressed, I was sick and needed help—not a pill." They also wanted her to see a psychologist or even a psychiatrist, but she knew that wouldn't solve her problems.

Finally, at one appointment, a doctor from Johns Hopkins took the time to sit with her and go over her medical file. "For the first time in

eight years," she said, "I had someone who truly cared and listened."
Luckily, Angie had just read our previous book, Could It Be B₁₂?
At her meeting with the Johns Hopkins doctor, Angie mentioned the
book. The doctor agreed that B₁₂ could explain her symptoms, and
ordered blood tests. Two days later Angie's doctor advised her to "start
on B₁₂ shots right away." Angie was deficient in both B₁₂ and iron,
and needed immediate treatment for both problems.

Soon after starting treatment, Angie felt a difference. Her hands
were no longer ice cold, and she had energy again. Her leg cramps
and dizzy spells lessened, and her cognitive symptoms began to fade.
After years of living in a fog, she can now think clearly again, and she
can plan for her future. "Now I am a foster parent," she says, "and
who knows—maybe I can have a child of my own someday."

The sad thing is that Angie's ordeal was completely preventable. She
didn't have "depression," and she didn't need medications or a psychi-
atrist. Initially, she needed a doctor who understood that she would
require lifelong supplementation with B₁₂ after her lap-band proce-
dure. And when that doctor failed her, she needed her other doctors to
recognize that her miscarriages, her psychological symptoms, and her
physical symptoms all stemmed from this terrible oversight.

———

WHAT DOCTORS DON'T KNOW ABOUT LOW B₁₂, B₁₂ DEFICIENCY, AND MENTAL ILLNESS

Why do so many doctors fail to give patients like Ricky, Brian, Matthew, and Angie the help they need? Because while increasing numbers of doctors are beginning to recognize that B₁₂ deficiency can cause psychiatric symptoms in the elderly, most still aren't aware that children, teens, and young adults who are B₁₂ deficient can develop these symptoms as well. But they frequently do, so it's not just your grandmother or your mother who may be at risk. It's also you—or your child. Here are some recent cases that show how B₁₂ can cause mental illness at any age.

- A 16-year-old girl became very anxious, stopped eating, and began having hallucinations. She became depressed, couldn't walk or sleep, had high blood pressure, and developed seizures. After speaking with the girl, doctors reported: "She did not respond to conversation; she could not answer the questions." Results of all lab tests were normal except for her serum B$_{12}$, which was extremely low. The doctors treated her solely with B$_{12}$ injections, and within one week her symptoms completely disappeared.[4]

- Doctors in Australia, evaluating a 21-year-old patient diagnosed with anxiety disorder and conversion disorder—a psychiatric diagnosis applied when doctors believe that a patient is converting emotional distress into physical symptoms, such as paralysis or blindness—discovered that she didn't have a psychiatric illness at all. She had a physical illness: B$_{12}$ deficiency, caused by her illegal use of "whipped cream bulbs" containing nitrous oxide. When the doctors gave her three injections of B$_{12}$, her neurological and psychiatric symptoms disappeared almost completely.[5]

- Doctors in London reported the case of a 27-year-old singer who stopped working, became withdrawn, and eventually became catatonic. "She was very slow to initiate movements," her doctors said, "took a long time to get out of bed, and would stand in the same position for long periods in the ward, often with her arms folded across her chest. She also followed members of staff around the ward repeating what they said. During an interview, she spent the whole time sitting in an erect posture in her chair with her hands clasped in a praying position." The doctors treated her with an antidepressant, but she did not respond. When lab tests showed a very low B$_{12}$ level, they started her on

4 M. Dogan et al., "Psychotic Disorder, Hypertension and Seizures Associated with Vitamin B$_{12}$ Deficiency: A Case Report," *Human & Experimental Toxicology* 31, no. 4 (April 2012): 410–13. DOI: 10.1177/0960327111422404. Epub 2011 Oct 25.
5 A. Brett, "Myeloneuropathy from Whipped Cream Bulbs Presenting as Conversion Disorder," *Australia and New Zealand Journal of Psychiatry* 31, no. 1 (1997): 131–2.

B_{12} injections. She improved rapidly (though she suffered another attack of catatonia when one B_{12} shot was delayed) and she is now out of the hospital, lives on her own, and is planning to enroll in a music course.[6]

- A 29-year-old woman with a history of obsessive-compulsive disorder went to her doctor complaining of anxiety. The woman intermittently took iron for her anemia and was taking Prozac for her psychological symptoms. The doctor's examination revealed that the woman had anxiety and mood swings, and her physical exam showed that she was very pale. Her blood work showed that her serum B_{12} and iron were extremely low.[7]

- A 62-year-old woman wound up in a psychiatric center after police found her wandering lost and confused. She was depressed and anxious, couldn't sleep, couldn't concentrate, and had trouble speaking. Tests revealed that she was suffering from delirium and depression, along with cognitive problems. Doctors discovered that her serum B_{12} was very low and began therapy. Two weeks after treatment started, her depression began to fade and she was able to think more clearly. Within four weeks of starting treatment, her depression and cognitive problems were totally gone, and she went back to working full time.[8]

> When low levels of B_{12} are the cause, a safe, simple cure exists and drugs are not needed.

- Another recent case involved a 64-year-old woman whose decline was so drastic that her doctors initially thought she had Creutzfeldt-Jakob disease (which is similar to "mad cow"

6 S. Jauhar et al., "Pernicious Anaemia Presenting as Catatonia without Signs of Anaemia or Macrocytosis," *British Journal of Psychiatry* 197, no. 3 (September 2010): 244–45. DOI: 10.1192/bjp.bp.108.054072.

7 A. B. Middleman and M. W. Melchiono, "A Routine CBC Leads to a Non-routine Diagnosis," *Adolescent Medicine* 7, no. 3 (1996): 423–26.

8 K. Mavrommati and O. Sentissi, "Delirium as a Result of Vitamin B_{12} Deficiency in a Vegetarian Female Patient," *European Journal of Clinical Nutrition* 67, no. 9 (September 2013): 996–97. DOI: 10.1038/ejcn.2013.128. Epub 2013 Jul 17.

disease). Over the course of two months, she became disoriented, lost her ability to pay attention to what was going on around her, and became unable to speak. She also had difficulty walking and had neck and shoulder pain. After getting a diagnosis of B$_{12}$ deficiency and undergoing three months of treatment, she recovered fully.[9]

Most of these adult patients were very lucky, because their B$_{12}$ deficiencies didn't last long enough to cause permanent damage. But the majority of patients with psychiatric symptoms related to low B$_{12}$ aren't so fortunate. All too often, doctors choose antidepressants, antianxiety drugs, or antipsychotics as first-line treatments for these patients' symptoms, allowing their underlying neurological damage to progress and eventually become irreversible.

These drugs can be very expensive, and quite dangerous. Serious, even fatal physical side effects have been reported, and they make a significant percentage of patients suicidal. While these medications are necessary for many patients, they *aren't* necessary when a patient has B$_{12}$ deficiency and a safe, simple cure exists.

Conversely, there is no downside to vitamin B$_{12}$ treatment. It's easy to administer and inexpensive, and even at the highest doses, it's completely harmless. Interestingly, some doctors report that psychotic symptoms that were resistant to psychotropic medications dramatically improved after B$_{12}$ therapy.[10,11,12] That's no surprise, since we know that B$_{12}$ plays a crucial role in neurotransmitter synthesis.

---

9 M. Payán Ortiz et al., "A Cyanocobalamin Deficiency That Simulates Creutzfeldt-Jakob Disease," *Neurologia*. 26, no. 5 (June 2011): 307–9. DOI: 10.1016/j.nrl.2010.12.016. Epub 2011 Feb 25.

10 G. Catalano et al., "Catatonia: Another Neuropsychiatric Presentation of Vitamin B$_{12}$ Deficiency?" *Psychosomatics* 39 (1998): 456–60.

11 R. Masalha et al., "Cobalamin-Responsive Psychosis as the Sole Manifestation of Vitamin B$_{12}$ Deficiency," *Israel Medical Association Journal* 3 (2001): 701–3.

12 D. Raveendranatan et al., "Vitamin B$_{12}$ Deficiency Masquerading as Clozapine-Resistant Psychotic Symptoms in Schizophrenia," *Journal of Neuropsychiatry and Clinical Neuroscience* 25 (2013): e34–e35.

———

Beverly worked for an insurance company. At age 37, she started suffering episodes of depression and mania. Doctors diagnosed her with bipolar disorder and treated her with prescription drugs, but the medications didn't help. At 42, Beverly finally wound up in the hospital in an agitated and suicidal state after losing large amounts of money at a casino.

Beverly's new doctors continued to treat her with medications, but the drugs had no effect. Over the next month, Beverly cycled between depressed and manic phases. She was agitated and distractible, experienced feelings of worthlessness, and believed she was about to suffer a catastrophe. She also behaved in a seductive manner, talked constantly, and couldn't sleep.

Over time, Beverly's symptoms grew even worse. She became confused and disoriented, and she developed delusions of persecution. Physical examinations revealed neurological problems, and results of an EEG were found to be abnormal as well.

At this point, doctors checked Beverly's serum B$_{12}$ and folate levels. Both were extremely low, and further tests showed that Beverly had pernicious anemia. The doctors gave Beverly B$_{12}$ injections and oral folate. She started responding within the first week of treatment and steadily improved over time. At a two-year follow-up, she showed no signs of mental illness.[13]

———

At 52 years of age, Suzanne gradually developed paralysis in her legs. Her doctor referred her to a neurologist, who diagnosed her with multiple sclerosis. Over the next two months, Suzanne was placed on numerous medications, but her leg weakness progressed and the drugs did not help. She required a cane, then used a walker, and eventually

13 M. Fafouti et al., "Mood Disorder with Mixed Features Due to Vitamin B(12) and Folate Deficiency," *General Hospital Psychiatry* 24, no. 2 (March–April 2002): 106–9.

needed a wheelchair to get around. As time went by, Suzanne became agitated and angry. She grew paranoid, and she called the police to report that her family was trying to poison her. She also became violent, throwing furniture and even trying to jump from a moving car.

Suzanne's family, stunned and frightened by her worsening behavior, finally took her to an emergency psychiatric center. She appeared disheveled, was delirious, disoriented, and paranoid, and could not stand without assistance. The psychiatric facility did a medical workup that included B$_{12}$ testing and found Suzanne to be profoundly deficient. Her serum B$_{12}$ was only 9 pg/mL.

The doctors diagnosed Suzanne with subacute combined degeneration of the spinal cord and psychosis due to a severe vitamin B$_{12}$ deficiency. Additional tests revealed that she suffered from autoimmune pernicious anemia.

Two days after starting B$_{12}$ injections, Suzanne started regaining the strength in her legs. Within eight weeks, symptoms of mental illness vanished. Unfortunately, she may never fully regain her health and mobility, because of her misdiagnosis.[14]

———

WHAT THE SCIENCE SHOWS

In addition to case reports, large-scale studies are revealing a close link between B$_{12}$ deficiency and psychiatric symptoms. In a 2013 paper, for instance, doctors reported a series of 19 patients who developed symptoms of mental illness as a result of B$_{12}$ deficiency. "A large number of our cases were diagnosed

> One study of psychiatric patients showed 20 percent had a vitamin B$_{12}$ deficiency.

with psychosis," they reported, with symptoms including hallucinations, delusions, and depression. Importantly, the majority of these patients did *not* have significant blood abnormalities or neurologic

14 G. Payinda and T. Hansen, "Vitamin B(12) Deficiency Manifested as Psychosis Without Anemia," *American Journal of Psychiatry* 157 (2000): 660–61.

symptoms such as pain or tingling in the extremities. The doctors say their finding "emphasizes the importance of investigation for vitamin B_{12} deficiency in psychiatrically ill patients, especially those in high-risk groups."[15]

In another recent study, clinicians screened 199 depressed patients and found that 73 had low-normal B_{12} levels. (Actually, many of the patients were not "low-normal" but overtly deficient by our standards.) The researchers divided the 73 patients with low B_{12} into two groups, treating 34 of them with B_{12} and a selective serotonin reuptake inhibitor (SSRI) and the remaining 39 with only an SSRI. At a three-month follow-up, 100 percent of the group whose treatment included B_{12} showed at least a 20 percent reduction in scores on a depression screening tool called the HAM-D. In contrast, only 69 percent of the medication-only group showed a 20 percent or greater reduction in HAM-D scores. The researchers concluded that "vitamin B_{12} supplementation with antidepressants significantly improved depressive symptoms in our cohort."[16]

(It's surprising that these researchers did not take part of the group and place them solely on B_{12} without the antidepressant. This could be because clinical guidelines recommend the use of SSRIs as a first-line treatment, or an institutional review board wouldn't approve the design, for similar reasons.)

In a third study, researchers reviewed laboratory data from psychiatric patients and also measured B_{12} levels in a random sampling of patients whose dietary habits were documented. They reported that 20 percent of the patients had vitamin B_{12} deficiency and 10 percent had levels indicating profound deficiency. "Our findings confirm that vitamin B_{12} deficiency is not uncommon in psychiatric patients, even when exposed to adequate nutrition," they say, adding, "The true prevalence may be even greater since low serum levels may underestimate the actual extent of vitamin B_{12} deficiency."[17]

15 N. Jayaram et al., "Vitamin B_{12} Levels and Psychiatric Symptomatology: A Case Series," *Journal of Neuropsychiatry and Clinical Neuroscience* 25, no. 2 (spring 2013).
16 E. U. Syed, M. Wasay, and S. Awan, "Vitamin B_{12} Supplementation in Treating Major Depressive Disorder: A Randomized Controlled Trial," *Open Neurology Journal* 15, no. 7 (November 2013): 44–48.
17 H. Silver, "Vitamin B_{12} Levels Are Low in Hospitalized Psychiatric Patients," *Israeli Journal of Psychiatry and Related Sciences* 37, no. 1 (2000): 41–45.

POSTPARTUM DEPRESSION/PSYCHOSIS

We seldom see patients coming into the emergency department (ED) complaining of postpartum depression, because these women typically seek help from their obstetricians or avoid seeking help at all. However, in our own practice, two patients presented to the ED for postpartum depression; both were on antidepressants and were found to be B$_{12}$ deficient. Their obstetricians never considered B$_{12}$ deficiency, yet these doctors didn't hesitate to prescribe antidepressants. One of the women was so desperate she intentionally crashed her car into a brick wall.

Physician G. Daynes reported many years ago that in his own practice as medical director of a hospital in South Africa, he successfully treated eight women whose postpartum psychosis stemmed from B$_{12}$ deficiency. (Postpartum psychosis is the disorder involved in the well-publicized case of Andrea Yates, who murdered her five children. It is also linked to many other suicides and murders.) His patients' recoveries led him to recommend that all women with postpartum psychosis receive large doses of B$_{12}$. "Where the postpartum psychosis is not primarily caused by lack of vitamin B$_{12}$, the giving of the preparation will do no harm," he noted, "so it seems to me that in all such cases it should be given as soon as possible."[18] (Again, we recommend testing patients *before* treatment is initiated. Screening both mother and child may save a life.)

Clearly, the research shows that B$_{12}$ deficiency is a major culprit in depression, dementia, and other mental disorders. But as the case studies in this chapter also show, many doctors are unaware of the connection between B$_{12}$ and mental illness. The financial cost of this knowledge gap is huge, and the cost in terms of human suffering is inestimable.

18 G. Daynes, "Cyanocobalamin in Postpartum Psychosis," *South African Medical Journal* 49, no. 34 (1975): 1373.

TAKING ACTION IF YOU SPOT SYMPTOMS

To protect yourself and your family, demand testing if you, your child, or anyone else in your family develops any of the symptoms listed at the end of this chapter. If a physician is reluctant to test you or your loved one, it may be necessary to consult other doctors to find one who is willing to order the tests.

And one more note: Adults need to be advocates not only for their children, but for their own parents and grandparents as well. The cognitive decline caused by B_{12} deficiency can look like learning disabilities or autism in kids, depression or anxiety in adults, or dementia in older adults. Regardless of your family member's age and diagnosis, be sure a doctor rules out B_{12} deficiency properly (see Chapter 11 for more information).

NEUROPSYCHIATRIC SYMPTOMS THAT CAN BE
ASSOCIATED WITH B_{12} DEFICIENCY

The following neuropsychiatric and/or psychological symptoms are among the most commonly seen in people with B_{12} deficiency:

- Confusion or disorientation
- Memory loss
- Depression
- Suicidal ideations
- Cognitive decline (foggy thinking)
- Poor concentration
- Learning disabilities
- Dementia
- Mania
- Anxiety
- Poor attention span
- Obsessive-compulsive behaviors

- Intellectual disabilities
- Paranoia
- Irritability
- Apathy
- Personality changes
- Inappropriate sexual behavior
- Delusions
- Hallucinations
- Violent or aggressive behavior
- Schizophrenic symptoms
- Sleep disturbances
- Insomnia
- Changes in taste, smell, vision, and sensory/motor function that can be mistaken for psychiatric problems.

10

No Laughing Matter: Nitrous Oxide and B_{12} Deficiency

At some point, nearly everyone needs to undergo surgery or a major dental procedure. While it's scary to go "under the knife," patients expect their surgeons, anesthesiologists, and dentists do their best to reduce the risks of complications. Unfortunately, this trust is often misplaced. That's because medical procedures involving nitrous oxide can lead to severe B_{12} deficiency, and few doctors or dentists are aware of this and take steps to prevent this dangerous problem.

Nitrous oxide (N_2O) is an anesthetic agent used millions of times a year to reduce pain and sedate patients during surgical, dental, and other medical procedures. You probably know this agent better as "laughing gas" because of its well-known ability to make you feel giddy.

Unfortunately, nitrous oxide has another unusual property: It inactivates B_{12}, thereby making it unusable. This can cause a functional deficiency in people whose stores are fair or low, potentially leading to serious or even fatal problems. If your B_{12} levels are adequate, N_2O use during surgery usually isn't dangerous, because your body can renew its stores of B_{12} within a few days. However, even people with normal B_{12} stores can get into trouble if they undergo long procedures. If your B_{12} levels are marginal, or if you have an overt deficiency, an undetected B_{12} malabsorption problem, or a *MTHFR* gene mutation, exposure to nitrous oxide can have devastating consequences.

———

Several years ago, doctors reported a case involving a 4-month-old infant who needed a routine surgery to correct craniosynostosis (a problem in which the bones of the skull fuse too early).

At the time of the surgery, everything appeared to go well. But soon afterward, the infant stopped smiling and playing, developed feeding problems, and became "floppy" and unresponsive. Eventually, she became so dehydrated that she needed emergency treatment.

In the hospital, magnetic resonance imaging (MRI) scans revealed brain atrophy. Tests showed that the infant's serum B$_{12}$ had dropped to life-threatening levels after the nitrous oxide used in her surgery severely worsened her undiagnosed B$_{12}$ deficiency. At the time her doctors reported her case, they could not predict whether she would ever fully recover.[1]

———

This child suffered because doctors exposed her to N$_2$O without discovering her preexisting B$_{12}$ deficiency. Yet her doctors followed standard procedure—because standard procedure doesn't include testing patients for B$_{12}$ deficiency before they undergo surgery using N$_2$O.

This probably surprises you if anyone in your family has had an operation, because doctors undoubtedly ordered an array of impressive-sounding tests beforehand: CBC, LYTES, RBS, BUN, CREAT, PT/PTT, UA, etc. Look at this list, however, and you'll find that serum B$_{12}$, the most basic test for B$_{12}$ deficiency, isn't on it. Neither is a urinary methylmalonic acid (MMA) assay, which often identifies B$_{12}$-deficient patients when the serum B$_{12}$ does not.

There is no excuse for this oversight, because nitrous oxide's ability to wreak havoc on the mind and body of a B$_{12}$-deficient patient isn't a new discovery. Doctors first reported the phenomenon more

1 J. K. McNeely et al., "Severe Neurological Impairment in an Infant after Nitrous Oxide Anesthesia," *Anesthesiology* 93 (2000: 1549–50).

than 35 years ago, and dozens of case studies are described in the medical literature. Moreover, it's not just a handful of patients who are at risk. Neurosurgeons Kathryn Holloway and Anthony Alberico say, "Because B_{12} deficiency is not uncommon and N_2O use is ubiquitous, the potential exists in every [surgical] practice for this complication to occur." Thus, they stress, "The surgeon should . . . look for evidence of B_{12} deficiency in every patient."[2] However, very few doctors follow this advice.

Why don't doctors, dentists, and oral surgeons test for B_{12} deficiency before a surgery? One reason is that most doctors assume, wrongly, that the standard presurgical complete blood count (CBC) will turn up any B_{12} problems (for more on this, see Chapter 11). The primary reason, however, is that many doctors and dentists simply aren't aware of the risks of administering N_2O to patients who are low or deficient in B_{12} and don't know that this anesthetic agent inactivates B_{12}. Moreover, even doctors who do know about N_2O's potential negative effects mistakenly think that bad reactions, as well as B_{12} deficiency itself, are extremely rare.

A small number of anesthesiologists do give patients a single injection of B_{12} before procedures involving N_2O, looking to reduce the risk of a dangerous reaction in anyone who might have low B_{12} stores. However, this "one-shot" approach probably won't prevent complications in severely deficient patients who are exposed to N_2O for several hours. It also makes no attempt to identify preoperative B_{12} deficiencies that will continue to cause insidious damage, and may even have contributed to the disorders that led to the need for a surgery or procedure in the first place. Also, giving an undiagnosed patient a single shot of B_{12} can cloud the results of future lab tests, leaving other doctors unable to identify a deficiency if one is lurking. Instead, doctors should follow the protocols we outline in Chapter 11, which provide clear instructions for determining if a deficiency exists.

---

2 K. Holloway and A. Alberico, "Postoperative Myeloneuropathy: A Preventable Complication in Patients with B_{12} Deficiency," *Journal of Neurosurgery* 72 (May 1990): 732–36.

How great is the risk for N$_2$O-related problems after surgery?

As we've noted, even doctors who are aware of N$_2$O's effects on B$_{12}$ think that problems are rare. However, the numbers tell a different story.

First, consider that U.S. hospitals perform more than 53 million surgical procedures each year, many involving N$_2$O—yet these hospitals screen only a handful of patients for B$_{12}$ deficiency. Dentists also perform millions of in-office surgical procedures each year, many of them involving N$_2$O. However, few if any check to determine if patients have a history of, are at risk for, or have signs and symptoms of B$_{12}$ deficiency. Some dentists even offer N$_2$O for dental cleanings.

Now, remember that overt B$_{12}$ deficiency (serum B$_{12}$ less than 200 pg/mL) is found in 3 percent of children under the age of 4, and low B$_{12}$ (which is commonly shown to be a real deficiency when MMA levels are measured) was not studied in this age group. (In Chapter 11 we detail the case of Jack, who had a serum B$_{12}$ level of 272 pg/mL. This was considered "normal," but MMA testing proved he had a profound deficiency.)

Overt B$_{12}$ deficiency is present in 3 percent of the adult U.S. population, and low B$_{12}$ levels exist in 15 percent of people between the ages of 20 and 59 (the statistics for seniors are even higher). This means that almost one in every five adult Americans is at risk if exposed to N$_2$O. We don't know the true incidence of children with low B$_{12}$ being exposed to N$_2$O, but it appears to be similar to adults—which is problematic.

Next, add in the fact that millions of people also have the *MTHFR* gene defect we discussed in Chapter 3, which may cause them to be more susceptible to low B$_{12}$. These people are at high risk for surgical complications if they're exposed to N$_2$O, even if their B$_{12}$ levels are normal before their surgeries. And they're in real trouble if their initial levels are suboptimal.

Finally, consider that children diagnosed with autism or other developmental disabilities receive N_2O frequently because they have difficulty being cooperative and holding still even for simple procedures such as dental cleanings. As we discussed in Chapter 8, many children diagnosed with autism or other developmental disabilities may actually have B_{12}-deficiency Acquired Brain Injury (BABI), which will worsen if these children are exposed to N_2O.

All of this—millions of high-risk patients, millions of surgeries using N_2O, and a virtual lack of B_{12} screening—creates a huge potential for serious, life-threatening side effects. Holloway and Alberico say, "It is tempting to speculate on how many unexpected new postoperative neurological deficits in surgical patients may have actually been due to B_{12} deficiency and nitrous oxide administration."[3]

But all we can do is speculate, because the issue has never been the subject of an in-depth epidemiologic investigation. Logic tells us, however, that for every patient diagnosed with obvious symptoms of B_{12} depletion due to N_2O, many more are likely to suffer symptoms that are wrongly written off as coincidental—especially since these symptoms may arise weeks or months after surgery.

RECREATIONAL N_2O AND B_{12} DEFICIENCY

In addition to its legitimate medical uses, N_2O is a popular recreational drug that is available through the Internet and at clubs. It's sold on the streets in whipped cream canisters or tanks, in balloons, or in small cartridges called "whippits." Young adults, teenagers, and even "tweens" are abusing N_2O in large numbers—and the practice is growing because the drug is easy to get.

"Huffing" N_2O is especially dangerous for individuals who are already low in B_{12}. However, it can cause severe symptoms even in people who have normal B_{12} levels when they begin abusing the drug. And the more frequently people abuse N_2O, the greater their risk becomes.

3 Ibid.

———

Sixteen-year-old Amanda arrived at the pediatric emergency department in big trouble. She was experiencing progressive numbness in her arms and legs, as well as sensory ataxia (meaning that she had relatively normal coordination when her eyes were open, but poor coordination when she closed them).

Amanda admitted to her doctor that she'd frequently inhaled nitrous oxide over the preceding three months in order to get high. Magnetic resonance imaging showed damage to her spinal cord (subacute combined degeneration) due to B$_{12}$ deficiency caused by N$_2$O abuse.[4]

———

Amanda's symptoms of numbness and ataxia are very common results of B$_{12}$ deficiency due to nitrous oxide abuse. Mental problems, including outright psychosis, can also occur. One case, for instance, involved a 33-year-old who believed he was part of an experiment for NASA and described himself as an "interface" between humans and machines. The man broke a window at home, destroyed furniture, and rode his bike into a moving car.[5]

Because N$_2$O is such a common recreational drug, it should be suspected as a culprit if a child, teen, or young adult develops psychiatric or neurological problems. Ask doctors to consider this possibility, even if the young person strongly denies using the drug.

SPOTTING SYMPTOMS OF B$_{12}$ DEFICIENCY DUE TO N$_2$O EXPOSURE

Clearly, the medical community needs to recognize the potential for either medical or illicit N$_2$O use to cause dangerous B$_{12}$ deficiency. But until they do, it's up to you to insist on B$_{12}$ testing before

4 M. H. Hu et al., "Nitrous Oxide Myelopathy in a Pediatric Patient," *Pediatric Emergency Care* 30, no. 4 (April 2014): 266–67.
5 N. K. Sethi et al., "Nitrous Oxide "Whippit" Abuse Presenting with Cobalamin Responsive Psychosis," *Journal of Medical Toxicology* 2, no. 2 (June 2006): 71–74.

any family member has a medical procedure involving nitrous oxide. (This is especially true if the procedure involves an infant, a child with autism or other developmental delays, or a person with any red flags for B_{12} deficiency.) And it's also up to you to keep a very close eye on your children when they reach the "tween" or teen years, and take immediate action if they show any symptoms that could stem from B_{12} deficiency due to illicit N_2O use.

The following symptoms can occur after surgery in patients with low B_{12} who received nitrous oxide. The same symptoms can occur in people who use nitrous oxide as a recreational drug. Note: These signs and symptoms have been mentioned in other chapters. However, with N_2O use or abuse, the symptoms of B_{12} deficiency may present acutely (swiftly, within days, weeks, or months), rather than slowly and insidiously. Remember, N_2O interferes with the B_{12} molecule and changes it to an inactive form not functional to the nervous system. Therefore, the serum B_{12} may be normal and homocysteine and MMA testing are needed (see Chapter 11 for more information).

Adults:

- Neuropathies (numbness or other abnormal sensations) or unexplained pains
- Depression
- Confusion or memory loss
- Dementia
- Difficulty walking
- Balance problems or falls
- Dizziness
- Transient ischemic attacks (TIAs)
- Strokes
- Fatigue
- Weakness
- Psychosis
- Suicidal or homicidal thoughts

Children:

- Developmental delay or regression
- Apathy
- Irritability
- Depression
- Anxiety
- Clumsiness
- Balance and/or gait problems
- Learning disabilities
- Behavioral changes
- Failure to thrive
- Weakness
- Fatigue
- Strokes
- Tremors
- Seizures
- In children already diagnosed with autism or other developmental delays, a worsening of symptoms

A RISING RISK

Medical professionals are using N_2O with increasing frequency for a variety of diagnostic procedures, especially those involving children. For example, here's an advertisement from a hospital using N_2O. You'll notice that there is no mention of screening for B_{12} deficiency and no mention of the potential dangers of using this anesthetic agent—or even preventative B_{12} treatment post-procedure.

Several years ago, Dr. Zier—a specialist in the pediatric intensive care unit at Children's Hospitals and Clinics of Minnesota—was waiting in her dentist's office for a routine teeth cleaning to start when she noticed a framed certificate for the dental hygienist's credentials to administer the gas nitrous oxide. Zier writes: "I thought, if a dental hygienist can give nitrous oxide to patients, why can't I? I knew we could use it for our patients at Children's."

The group introduced nitrous oxide at Children's in 2004. This innovation makes Children's the only nurse-administered nitrous oxide program in the United States. Nitrous oxide is now used for some procedures at Children's. . . . Many children receive it when they undergo a radiological test of the urinary system. . . . Other children receive nitrous oxide when they need a needle inserted for an intravenous line or for nuclear medicine procedures involving a catheter and fluids.[6]

Other institutions are following suit, without understanding how this practice can cause or contribute to B_{12} deficiency in children. Here is a case in point. In June 2014, a nurse I work with relayed that her son was being worked up for autism and was sedated with N_2O so he would lie still during a brain MRI. His doctors did not mention the effect of N_2O on vitamin B_{12} in the body, nor did they test or treat the child before or after the procedure. Oversights like this are clear evidence that health-care professionals are simply unaware of the physiology of B_{12} and nitrous oxide.

6 S. Thompson, "I had a dream—a good dream!" Children's Hospitals and Clinics of Minnesota website, www.childrensmn.org/web/whatsnew/097261.asp (February 11, 2009).

11

Taking Charge: Preventing or Identifying a B$_{12}$ Deficiency in Your Child

In this book, we've introduced you to many victims of the epidemic of B$_{12}$ deficiency. These victims include babies who became developmentally disabled for life, children and teens who developed learning and social disabilities or lost their ability to walk, mothers who became too physically or mentally crippled to care for their children, and many others whose lives were interrupted or even destroyed by this stealthy attacker.

We know that these stories are frightening. But here's the most important lesson we want you to learn from them: *You can protect yourself and everyone in your family from this crippling disorder.* B$_{12}$ deficiency is one medical condition that is entirely preventable; it is relatively simple to treat, and when it is detected in its early stages, prompt supplementation can lead to complete reversal of symptoms. Even in the later stages of a deficiency, remarkable improvement is sometimes possible.

To protect your family, however, you need to have all the facts. In this chapter, we tie it all together and provide you with a plan of action. We explain how to prevent B$_{12}$ deficiency, how to detect its possible signs, how to ensure that your doctor orders the correct tests to determine if a deficiency exists, and how to get proper treatment if tests reveal a problem. In addition, we provide information on tests and treatments that you can show to your physician.

———

Jack, a 10-month-old baby, had spina bifida occulta and a tethered spinal cord and was scheduled for surgery. Nancy, Jack's grandmother, had read the first edition of Could It Be B$_{12}$? *and asked Jack's mother Kelly to read the information on N$_2$O.*

After reading the chapter and speaking with us, Kelly had Jack tested for B$_{12}$ deficiency because of his poor head growth and developmental delays. She was concerned as well about the upcoming surgery, and verified that it would indeed involve nitrous oxide.

Kelly sent Jack's urine sample to Norman Clinical Laboratory, Inc., where testing showed that his urinary MMA was grossly elevated, indicating a true vitamin B$_{12}$ deficiency. The chief of neurosurgery postponed Jack's spinal surgery, agreeing that "B$_{12}$ deficiency must be addressed and can lead to neurological complications."

Despite this, several pediatric specialists—a pediatrician, two neurologists, a gastroenterologist, two hematologists and two geneticists—denied Jack B$_{12}$ treatment because it wasn't "normal" protocol. Their response made no sense; it's as if they were so unfamiliar with this medical condition that they were afraid to take responsibility for treating Jack, with each specialist wanting another to take the lead. Kelly tried to educate them, but to no avail—although they all acknowledged that B$_{12}$ treatment is harmless.

Kelly said, "I was told nothing was wrong with my son, and that we should take no action. I was told head measurement varies and is subjective, and development varies in children. I was told that Jack's level of B$_{12}$ (257 pg/mL) was within the normal range and that since he was not anemic and did not have megaloblastic cells, he did not have a B$_{12}$ deficiency. I was told his elevated urinary MMA of 26.4 µmol/L (normal <3.8) was only an indicator of [a metabolic condition called] methylmalonic aciduria. All of which is, unfortunately, completely wrong. I was made to feel like an overly worried mother, given all the doctors noted that Jack was a 'happy baby' and said 'calm down, Mom.'" Repeat MMA testing (now using blood) from a *different laboratory ordered by Jack's doctors still showed his deficiency—serum MMA of 8.0 μmol/L (normal <0.04 μmol/L).*

We encouraged Kelly to begin treatment on her own while she searched for a doctor willing to give Jack B_{12} (hydroxocobalamin) injections. Kelly began giving Jack high-dose methylcobalamin lozenges daily, dissolving the tablet in a small amount of milk and feeding it to him. A few months later, Kelly found another pediatric gastroenterologist who determined that Jack did indeed have a B_{12} deficiency and was willing to treat Jack with B_{12} injections. Post-treatment, Jack's levels of serum B_{12} increased and his urinary methylmalonic acid decreased to normal levels, making the B_{12} deficiency diagnosis conclusive.

Kelly noticed that the hydroxocobalamin injections resulted in significant improvement compared to the methylcobalamin lozenges. Jack received 10 (1,000-mcg) injections every other day. "Prior to the tenth shot," Kelly said, "I hadn't seen much of a difference—but then on the tenth visit to get the shot, Jack pointed to a picture in the room [he hadn't been pointing], and he waved when the nurse left the room [he hadn't been waving]." Previously, Jack was not able to hold a phone up to his ear, but now he could. Jack had been in physical therapy, and at the next assessment, after his series of B_{12} injections, he met all his milestones. He had been behind on all of them previously.

After Jack began B_{12} treatment, his head growth accelerated and his head circumference climbed from the 8th to the 25th percentile. Unfortunately, Jack's new pediatric gastroenterologist decided at this point that Jack didn't need B_{12} treatment anymore. "From there," Kelly says, "I watched his head circumference drop again." It had been at the 35th percentile of normal at birth, dropping to the 8th percentile before B_{12} treatment began. After treatment, it rose to the 25th percentile but then dropped off again to the 16th percentile when treatment stopped. "During the drop," Kelly says, "I again approached his doctors to continue his treatment with B_{12}. No one would. That was when I took matters into my own hands and began putting methyl-B_{12} into his bottles of milk."

Along the way, a doctor did end up prescribing intermittent B₁₂ shots. Then Kelly placed Jack back on high-dose oral methyl-B₁₂. Overall, since about 1 year of age, with some on-and-off periods early on, Jack has had a minimum of at least 1,000 mcg of oral methyl-B₁₂ per day.

Jack's spinal operation was a success, and he experienced no postoperative complications. Luckily, Kelly was armed with the information in our book. She said, "I have no doubt that without this book, and the information therein, my son would now be mentally retarded, and might be suffering from neurological damage, and even autistic behaviors."

By the time he was 5 years old, Jack met all his physical milestones according to his physical therapist, and his mental development was also right on track. Kelly reports, "Later, after Jack turned five, I was working more and also relaxed a little, and I got a bit distracted and lazy about giving him B₁₂. I also thought he might not need it as much. That was when we noticed that Jack developed uncontrollable neurological tics (sniffing, blinking, or clearing his throat constantly). I discovered that when he went back on B₁₂, within days to a few weeks, the tics would reduce in frequency and then would go away. Over time, I realized there was no mistake—the B₁₂ was keeping the tics away." Further testing showed that Jack, Kelly, and Jack's dad all have a MTHFR mutation.

Today, at the age of 9, Jack has a high IQ of 139. His head size is slightly small and he needs to take B₁₂ (accompanied by folate) or he develops tics. Otherwise, he has no remaining problems. His mom reports, "At every conference with teachers, they say he is a delight. He has good friends, and plays basketball and soccer. I am so grateful to report that he is a happy, healthy, normal kid!"

B₁₂ treatment has made all the difference. Jack had been headed for a neurological injury and permanent intellectual disability—a tragic outcome prevented only by his mother's determination and the good fortune that put our book in her mother-in-law's hands.

Jack dodged a big bullet, but it wasn't due to his doctors' diligence. It was due to his mother's. Kelly adds, "Without my knowledge of B$_{12}$'s importance, Jack wouldn't have all the opportunities he has now to live a very full, normal, and happy life! And, instead of attending Battle of the Books competitions and basketball games, we'd be in physical, speech, and occupational therapies. It makes me angry to think back how specialist after specialist dismissed the clinical signs, and wouldn't treat Jack—but more than being angry, I am both scared and grateful—scared for all of the children out there who aren't fortunate enough to have Sally's book and counsel, and grateful that we had it so that I could protect my son from this kind of preventable injury."

PROTECT YOUR FAMILY BY BEING PROACTIVE

There are two ways to protect your family from the terrible consequences of B$_{12}$ deficiency. The first, and obviously the best, is to make sure a deficiency doesn't occur at all. When this isn't possible, the next-best thing is to ensure that a doctor identifies and treats a deficiency before it does any additional damage. Here are the steps you can take to prevent a deficiency or find out if one already exists.

> If you decide that you or someone in your family should be tested for B$_{12}$ deficiency, DO NOT start administering B$_{12}$ supplements before the tests are performed.

SPOT POSSIBLE SYMPTOMS AND RED FLAGS

In previous chapters, we've outlined the most common symptoms of B$_{12}$ deficiency in different age groups, as well as symptoms seen in people with inborn errors of B$_{12}$ metabolism. Review those symptoms and red flags for at-risk patients, or see the Appendices at the back of this book.

If you spot symptoms of B$_{12}$ deficiency in yourself or another family member, or if you identify red flags that put someone in your family at risk for a deficiency, communicate your concerns to your doctor immediately and ask for testing (see Appendix H).

One important note: If you decide that you or someone in your family should be tested for B$_{12}$ deficiency, *do not start administering B$_{12}$ supplements before the tests are performed.* This will skew the results, possibly convincing the doctor that the person is perfectly fine when low B$_{12}$ or a deficiency actually exists. In addition, patients pursuing a malpractice case due to chronic misdiagnosis and injury will have a case only if they have laboratory documentation to prove a deficiency existed.

GUARD AGAINST B$_{12}$ DEFICIENCY IN VEGETARIANS AND VEGANS

If any of your family members are vegetarians or vegans, or eat a macrobiotic diet, it's crucial to supplement their diets with vitamin B$_{12}$. We recommend at least 1,000 mcg daily using sublingual supplements, sometimes called oral lozenges. We recommend methyl-B$_{12}$, adenosyl-B$_{12}$, or hydroxo-B$_{12}$ rather than cyano-B$_{12}$. Sublingual B$_{12}$ supplements can be purchased at a variety of health food stores, pharmacies, or supermarkets without a prescription. There are many reputable over-the-counter active B$_{12}$ products. Two brands we personally have used and recommend are Superior Source Vitamins and NOW Foods.

Be careful and knowledgeable about vegetarian foods being touted as high in B$_{12}$. Many vegetarians supplement their diets with spirulina (an algae), tempeh (fermented soy), or nori (a seaweed) in the belief that these plant foods contain vitamin B$_{12}$, a widely accepted idea based on laboratory tests that showed a certain amount of the vitamin in these plants. Research, however, shows that the tests are primarily detecting "pseudo-vitamin B$_{12}$" analogues that may actually block the uptake of real B_{12}.[1] In addition, these sources contain very low amounts of B_{12} in general and should not be used or relied on during pregnancy and breastfeeding.

This information has been known for decades, but somehow is still being ignored or misrepresented in many books and websites. As a result, it is not well understood in the vegan/vegetarian community, as this next case demonstrates.

———

Twenty-six-year-old Kate, a lacto-ovo vegetarian, decided to breastfeed her baby, Alex. She switched to a mostly vegan diet when Alex was 6 weeks old, because she found that eating dairy upset his digestion and caused eczema. This dietary change cleared up Alex's skin condition, and Kate's doctor assured her that Alex would be able to tolerate dairy and other foods when his digestion matured. Kate supplemented her diet with seaweed, barley grass, and chlorella, believing that these would provide adequate B_{12}. Alex reached all the typical milestones at the same time as his peers and was reported to be a happy, lively, content, and thriving baby.

In December 2013, 15-month-old Alex started rejecting solid food, began looking very pale, and became unusually tired. Kate took him to the pediatrician, asking to have his blood checked to see if he was deficient in iron (the only type of anemia she knew of). Her doctor assured her that Alex did not appear malnourished and was highly unlikely to be anemic. He said the blood tests would be far too traumatic.

Alex was breastfeeding well, and Kate began to breastfeed him more frequently to compensate for his refusal to eat solids. A few days later, the visiting nurse dropped by, and Kate asked for her advice. The nurse was alarmed by Alex's appearance and called the hospital. The nurse confirmed that Alex's weight was within normal range, but

1 F. Watanabe et al., "Pseudovitamin B(12) is the Predominant Cobamide of an Algal Health Food, Spirulina Tablets," *Journal of Agricultural and Food Chemistry* 47, no. 11 (1999): 4736–41.

was concerned that he was severely anemic. She urged Kate to take Alex to the emergency room.

Alex was admitted to the pediatric ward, where doctors determined that he was indeed very anemic and severely B_{12}-deficient. His serum B_{12} was only 30 pg/mL and his iron stores were low. Alex was given formula feedings through a nasogastric tube for four days. He did not improve with the tube feedings, and on day four of his admission, B_{12} injections were administered. Kate reported that within a few hours of receiving his first B_{12} injection, Alex's mood and behavior dramatically changed. He was able to eat again without any difficulties, interacted happily, and cruised around energetically. Alex was kept in the hospital for two weeks, and wasn't discharged home until he was drinking all his formula and eating two meat meals and two snacks every day.

Mom and child are back home now, and Alex appears to be thriving. However, the hospital called social services upon Alex's admission to the hospital to determine if a child protection plan needed to be put into action. Kate was put under investigation and had to meet with a social worker.

We fully understand the hospital's position, because Alex's doctors and nurses were concerned that he was not receiving adequate nutrition from a vegan breastfeeding mother. The hospital staff was responsible for ensuring his safety and was required to contact social services to intervene. There have been cases where vegetarian or vegan women refused to believe that their diet lacked the proper nutrients to sustain the health of their children, and these children suffered the consequences. (Some babies have died.)

The matter was resolved after proper investigation. Kate was educated regarding her diet and breastfeeding, and she explained that she thought she was properly supplementing with B_{12}.

Alex was also low in iron and zinc. His first pediatrician admitted that Kate had brought Alex to him concerned that he was anemic. It wasn't that Kate failed to seek medical attention. Instead, Kate was unaware of the dangers of breastfeeding while eating a vegan/vegetarian *diet, and was also unaware of the poor B_{12} content in the supplements she was taking. The first pediatrician failed both Alex and Kate by not inquiring about Kate's dietary history, or, if he did, by not anticipating B_{12} deficiency and guiding her properly. In addition, he did not work up Alex for anemia, even when Kate requested this.*

Fortunately, Alex responded quickly to proper treatment. But only time will tell if he will have any neurological deficits as a result of his brain being deprived of vitamin B_{12} during a critical period of growth and development.

———

We can't overemphasize the importance of correctly supplementing a vegetarian or vegan diet with B_{12}. As we've noted, the vast majority of long-term vegans are B_{12}-deficient, as are about a quarter of vegetarians. While a properly supplemented meat-free diet can be healthful, an improperly supplemented one can be extremely dangerous, especially to a growing fetus, infant, or young child—so don't take any chances.

GET FAMILY MEMBERS TESTED BEFORE ANY SURGERY INVOLVING N2O

In Chapter 10, we explained how the common anesthetic agent nitrous oxide (N_2O) inactivates vitamin B_{12}, putting patients exposed to this agent at risk for B_{12} deficiency or making an existing deficiency worse.

If you, your child, or another family member will be undergoing surgery or a dental procedure, ask if it will involve nitrous oxide. Any child with a developmental delay, neurological disorder, mental illness, or autism spectrum diagnosis should receive proper B_{12} testing (including MMA) before a procedure involving N_2O. If testing indicates low B_{12} or a deficiency, have the surgery postponed until the deficiency is addressed. This also applies to adults with symptoms of B_{12} deficiency or any significant risk factors.

We recommend that anyone receiving N$_2$O be given high-dose sublingual B$_{12}$[2] or a standard 1,000 mcg injection before and after the procedure. Be aware, too, that many anesthesiologists use N$_2$O during emergency C-sections. If you undergo an emergency C-section, insist on receiving high-dose B$_{12}$ afterward—especially if you will be breastfeeding.

TREAT *MTHFR* GENE MUTATIONS

MTHFR gene mutations, which we talked about in Chapter 3, are genetic variants that cause a key enzyme in the body to function at a lower rate than normal. This can lead to a variety of medical problems. There are more than 50 known *MTHFR* gene variants, but the two most well known and studied variants are C677T and A1298C (the numbers refer to their locations on the gene).

As we explained earlier, possessing homozygous C677T or the compound heterozygous mutation will reduce your body's ability to use B$_{12}$ and folate. Individuals who have known *MTHFR* gene mutations need to take the active forms of folate (levomefolic acid, 5-MTHF, L-methylfolate, and 5-methyltetrahydrofolate) and the active forms of vitamin B$_{12}$ (methylcobalamin and adenosylcobalamin) to compensate for this.

A variety of over-the-counter products are available, as well as prescription vitamins and nutrients that contain the active forms of folic acid and B$_{12}$. Additional supplements used to augment the methylation pathway are betaine, S-adenosylmethionine (SAMe), and trimethylglycine (TMG). If B$_{12}$ injections are used, they should contain methylcobalamin or hydroxocobalamin, not cyanocobalamin. The advantage of hydroxocobalamin is that it can be easily converted to both active forms of B$_{12}$.

People with *MTHFR* gene mutations can have falsely normal and/or elevated serum B$_{12}$ levels, which is why MMA and Hcy testing can also help diagnose these patients.

---

2 High-dose oral or sublingual B$_{12}$ means 1,000 micrograms (mcg) or greater.

If defective *MTHFR* genes are an issue for anyone in your family, we strongly recommend that you consult with a knowledgeable doctor or nutritionist. Taking the correct supplements can lower your family member's risk of stroke, cancer, and other life-threatening conditions. Pregnant women or women wanting to conceive should be tested by their doctor to determine if they have a *MTHFR* gene defect, because if they do, they need to be on special prenatal vitamins.

UNDERSTANDING B_{12} TESTS

There are four tests that can help your doctor identify a B_{12} deficiency. One test measures levels of B_{12} (both active and inactive) in the blood, two tests measure other substances related to B_{12}, and the final test measures only active B_{12} in the blood.

The four tests are:

1. Serum B_{12}

2. Methylmalonic acid (MMA)—urine or blood

3. Homocysteine (Hcy)

4. Holotranscobalamin II (HoloTC or Active B_{12}).

Generally, doctors test for B_{12} deficiency using only the first test. We recommend that the first two tests be used together, especially when children are being tested. Research still needs to ascertain if the urinary MMA is more sensitive than the serum MMA. The remaining two tests may also be necessary in some cases. Here's a quick explanation of each test.

SERUM B_{12}

This test measures the level of vitamin B_{12} in your blood serum. It's cheap and easy, but it has three major drawbacks.

First, because this test measures inactive as well as biologically active B_{12}, it can yield falsely high results when levels of active B_{12} are actually low. Second, there's a great deal of controversy as to what constitutes a normal result for this test. While many doctors consider 200 pg/mL (picograms per milliliter) to be acceptable, we and many other experts believe that the normal serum B$_{12}$ threshold needs to be raised from 200 pg/mL to 500 pg/mL. We define this range (200 pg/mL to 500 pg/mL) as the *gray zone*. Patients who are symptomatic and whose B$_{12}$ is below 500 pg/mL need to be treated. *Both children and adults should have B$_{12}$ levels of 1,000 pg/mL or greater.*

Finally, researchers recently reported that newer serum B$_{12}$ tests, called competitive-binding luminescence assays, miss more than a third of true pernicious anemia (PA) cases. (PA, an autoimmune disorder, is the most well-known form of B$_{12}$ deficiency.) Up to 35 percent of saved samples from confirmed PA patients revealed false normal results using three different assays.[3] Because of the limitations of the serum B$_{12}$ test, this test should be used in conjunction with the MMA test described below if a patient is symptomatic or at risk.

Methylmalonic acid (MMA)

Vitamin B$_{12}$ is a cofactor for two necessary metabolic reactions. The first reaction involves adenosyl-B$_{12}$, which needs to be present in this form for the conversion of MMA to succinic acid. A B$_{12}$ deficiency impairs this pathway, causing MMA levels to build up. Thus, elevation of MMA typically indicates a B$_{12}$ deficiency.

Homocysteine (Hcy)

The second essential metabolic reaction in which vitamin B$_{12}$ is a cofactor involves methyl-B$_{12}$. B$_{12}$ must be present in the methyl form for the conversion of homocysteine to methionine to occur. As we discussed in Chapter 3, homocysteine can be recycled into methionine or converted into cysteine with the aid of vitamins B$_{12}$, B$_9$, and B$_6$. If you are deficient in any of these vitamins, homocysteine will accumulate in your body (blood and urine).

3 R. Carmel, *New England Journal of Medicine* 367 (2012): 1569–71. DOI: 10.1056/NEJMc1210169. Epub 2012 Oct 18

The Hcy test measures the level of homocysteine in the plasma. Elevated levels of Hcy can indicate vitamin B_{12}, vitamin B_9, or vitamin B_6 deficiency, but can occur in other medical conditions as well (e.g., dehydration, hypothyroidism, and renal insufficiency or failure).

This is a useful test (along with MMA) for symptomatic B_{12} patients who have been exposed to nitrous oxide during surgery, or patients known or suspected to have abused N_2O. Nitrous oxide interferes with the B_{12} molecule and changes it to an inactive form that is not useful to the nervous system but is measured by the serum B_{12} test; thus, the serum B_{12} can falsely indicate that B_{12} levels are normal in an N_2O-exposed patient. In this case, the Hcy and MMA tests can reveal a deficiency.

The Hcy test isn't necessary to diagnose B_{12} deficiency in most cases. However, it's a valuable adjunct to the serum B_{12} test because it can indicate if you're at elevated risk of vascular disease. Elevated levels may also be due to a *MTHFR* gene mutation and therefore merit investigation.

A NOTE FOR PEOPLE WITH VASCULAR DISEASE

People with vascular disease should always have their Hcy, MMA, serum B_{12}, and folate levels measured to determine if B vitamin deficiencies are causing or contributing to their health problems. These people may have a *MTHFR* or cystathionine beta synthase (CBS) defect and need proper evaluation and treatment.

Holotranscobalamin (HoloTC or active B_{12})

Only around 20 percent of total serum B_{12} is in the active form our bodies can use. This active B_{12}, called *HoloTC*, is bound to transcobalamin II, a transport protein. Because the HoloTC test only detects this active B_{12}, it is thought to be more sensitive than a serum B_{12} test. The HoloTC test has been available for decades, but was classified as investigational until recently.

Additional tests to know about

When a patient is severely or chronically B_{12} deficient, all three of the common tests (serum B_{12}, MMA, and Hcy) will typically agree. The serum B_{12} will be low, while the MMA and Hcy will be elevated. This scenario typically occurs when a patient is being diagnosed in the later stages of B_{12} deficiency, in which injury may have already occurred.

When doctors do identify a B_{12} deficiency, additional tests are often necessary to identify the underlying cause of the deficiency. Here are some tests your doctor may order, along with the medical conditions they can aid in identifying:

- Gastrin: autoimmune pernicious anemia (PA), atrophic gastritis (AG)

- Pepsinogen: AG

- Parietal cell antibody: PA

- Intrinsic factor antibody: PA

- *H. pylori* antibody test, urea breath test: *Helicobacter pylori* infection

- Tissue transglutaminase antibodies (IgG, IgA): celiac disease (gluten enteropathy)

- C-xylose breath test: small intestinal bacterial overgrowth

- MTHFR-2: *MTHFR* gene mutation

- Esophagogastroduodenoscopy (EGD): AG, gastric tumors

- Small intestinal biopsy: celiac disease

How to get proper treatment for your child

As we've noted above, we believe that any symptomatic patient in the "gray zone" (serum B_{12} 200 pg/mL to 500 pg/mL) should receive treatment. If you fall into this category, talk with your doctor about the different forms of B_{12} therapy. As we explain in the next chapter, we prefer injectable hydroxocobalamin or methylcobalamin to cyanocobalamin. We also prefer injected B_{12} to oral supplements. Regarding lozenges or sublingual B_{12}, we prefer methyl-B_{12}, adenosyl-B_{12}, and hydroxo-B_{12} over cyano-B_{12}. Nasal

> Make sure you continue your treatment for as long as necessary. Only a few causes of B_{12} deficiency are temporary.

sprays are similar in efficacy to oral and sublingual treatment, but keep in mind that prescription nasal B_{12} is cyanocobalamin. Transdermal patches are widely available but their efficacy has not been adequately studied.

No matter which form of treatment you receive, make sure that your treatment continues as long as necessary. A few causes of B_{12} deficiency are temporary. Many, however, are permanent, and taking extra B_{12} for only a few weeks or months won't solve the problem. If you have one of these conditions, you'll need to take supplemental B_{12} for life, and it's both your responsibility and your doctor's to make sure that there's no break in your treatment.

Sometimes doctors order serum B_{12} tests for patients who've undergone long-term B_{12} treatment, or are on current B_{12} therapy, in order to demonstrate to these patients that they're not deficient any longer—or even to convince them that they never suffered from a deficiency in the first place. This is misguided, because people who've been correctly treated for B_{12} deficiency will have good or even high serum B_{12} levels, and these levels will stay adequate for months or years once treatment is stopped. Eventually, however, the deficiency will return—and, with it, the risk of debilitating symptoms, injury, or even death.

In other cases, problems arise when patients switch to new doctors who aren't knowledgeable about B_{12} deficiency. We recommend that patients who receive a diagnosis of B_{12} deficiency obtain their test results and medical records and give copies of these to any new doctors. A physician who's skeptical about your assertion that you're B_{12}-deficient is more likely to listen to you if you have the documentation to prove it.

12

Testing and Treatment: Information for Physicians and Health-care Providers

While we've written this book primarily for medical consumers, we know that many physicians and other health-care professionals will be reading it as well. So in this chapter, we'd like to address some of the questions we hear most often from colleagues in the health-care community.

WHICH PATIENTS SHOULD UNDERGO SCREENING FOR B_{12} DEFICIENCY?

After years of clinical experience, as well as an extensive review of the literature, we developed the Cobalamin Deficiency Risk (CDR) Score in 1999 as a screening tool for doctors and other health-care providers. The CDR's point system allows clinicians to estimate a patient's relative risk of B_{12} deficiency. The CDR Score is for adults and has been updated for 2014. We have also created the Pediatric Cobalamin Deficiency Risk (PCDR) Score for neonates, infants, and children up to 18 years of age. These diagnostic tools are available in Appendices A and B, and can also be accessed from our website, **www.B12Awareness.org**.

WHICH TESTS SHOULD BE ORDERED?

The standard serum B_{12} test is useful, but physicians need to be aware that it fails to identify many patients with low cobalamin levels. For example, patients with underlying liver disease, alcoholism, myeloproliferative disorders, lymphoma, or small intestinal bacterial overgrowth often have falsely elevated serum B_{12} levels.

Also, there are serious questions about the accuracy of the newer competitive-binding luminescence assays (CBLA). These assays have replaced the older microbiologic and radioisotope-dilution assays, which had an accuracy of about 95 percent. Only a few studies have compared the CBLA's sensitivity and specificity with previous methods. The authors of one such study note that their results "suggest widespread malfunction" of the CBLA. These newer assays may show falsely elevated serum B$_{12}$ in patients who have autoantibodies against intrinsic factor.[1]

Additionally, we believe that the lower limit for the serum B$_{12}$ test currently is far too low. If patients are symptomatic and their serum B$_{12}$ falls in the gray zone (200–500 pg/mL), treatment needs to be initiated. Studies show that deficiencies begin to appear when B$_{12}$ levels in the cerebral spinal fluid are below 550 pg/mL.[2,3,4]

Another concern regarding the serum B$_{12}$ test is that only around 20 percent of total serum B$_{12}$ is bound to Transcobalamin II—the biologically active protein that transports B$_{12}$ throughout the body. The remaining B$_{12}$ (80 percent) is bound to Transcobalamin I and III and thus is inactive or biologically unavailable, but is still included in the total serum B$_{12}$ result, falsely elevating serum B$_{12}$ values.

When it comes to B$_{12}$ deficiency, many physicians tend to treat the number rather than the patient, which is a grave mistake, given the limitations of the serum B$_{12}$ test. Many times in our experience, a symptomatic patient with serum B$_{12}$ levels between 200 pg/mL and 350 pg/mL was told by the doctor: "You do not have a B$_{12}$ deficiency." Given the remarkable safety of B$_{12}$ treatment and the horrific consequences of ignoring a deficiency, it is always best to

1 R. Carmel, *New England Journal of Medicine* 367 (2012): 1569–71. DOI: 10.1056/NEJMc1210169. Epub 2012 Oct 18 .DOI: 10.1056/NEJMc1210169

2 C. J. M. VanTiggelen et al., "Assessment of Vitamin-B$_{12}$ Status in CSF," *American Journal of Psychiatry* 141, no. 1 (1984): 136–37.

3 Y. Mitsuyama and H. Kogoh, "Serum and Cerebrospinal Fluid Vitamin B$_{12}$ Levels in Demented Patients with CH3-B$_{12}$ Treatment—Preliminary Study," *Japanese Journal of Psychiatry and Neurology* 42, no. 1 (1988): 65–71.

4 C. J. M. VanTiggelen, J. P. C. Peperkamp, and J. F. W. TerToolen, "Vitamin-B$_{12}$ Levels of Cerebrospinal Fluid in Patients with Organic Mental Disorder," *Journal of Orthomolecular Psychiatry* 12 (1983): 305–11.

THE FATAL ERROR OF RELYING ON BLOOD ABNORMALITIES

In general, doctors considering a diagnosis of B_{12} deficiency are trained only to look for blood abnormalities in a complete blood count (CBC)—that is, anemia and, in particular, macrocytosis. However, nervous system symptoms often precede classic blood abnormalities by many years, and the neurological damage that underlies them can be permanent by the time macrocytosis appears.

Also, high levels of folic acid can make CBC results appear normal, even when a B_{12} deficiency exists. Clinicians often may not see macrocytosis or anemia in B_{12}-deficient patients because many countries have fortified their grains, cereals, and other foods with folic acid. This masking effect can also occur in patients taking over-the-counter supplements and prenatal vitamins. In addition, blood transfusions from healthy donors as well as prescription folic acid therapy can improve macrocytosis and/or anemia. So it's crucial to order B_{12} tests before prescribing folic acid therapy (e.g., prenatal vitamins) or before ordering a blood transfusion.

B_{12} deficiency often coexists with iron deficiency and can accompany other microcytic anemias. In these cases, a clinician may fail to suspect B_{12} deficiency because the patient will not have an elevated mean corpuscular volume. Don't be fooled by the CBC when ruling out B_{12} deficiency.

err on the side of treatment. Often, symptomatic patients whose serum B_{12} is in the gray zone are proven to have a B_{12} deficiency when other B_{12} markers are measured.

While raising the lower limit for B_{12} is one step in addressing a developing B_{12} deficiency, we also want to be clear that there are times when the additional markers for B_{12} deficiency (urinary MMA, Hcy, HoloTC) are needed. As a general rule, we advocate treating all patients who are symptomatic and have serum B_{12} levels under 500 pg/mL, regardless of the MMA, Hcy, and HoloTC results. In addition, symptomatic patients with "normal" serum B_{12}

but elevated urinary/serum MMA or Hcy, and/or low HoloTC require treatment. Children with developmental delay, cerebral palsy, or suspected autism need to receive the MMA and serum B$_{12}$ tests, as well as MTHFR-2 and cystathionine beta synthase genetic testing. And therapeutic trials should still be provided for symptomatic patients, even if blood/urine results are within the reference range.

Based on two decades of clinical experience, we believe that serum B$_{12}$ levels need to be 1,000 pg/mL or more for healthy brain growth and development in infants and children. We recommend the same level for optimal brain and nervous system health and prevention of disease in adults.

WHAT IS THE APPROPRIATE TREATMENT FOR B$_{12}$ DEFICIENCY?

There are four forms of supplemental vitamin B$_{12}$: cyanocobalamin, hydroxocobalamin, methylcobalamin, and adenosylcobalamin. Different recommendations exist for initial and maintenance therapy. Here is the most commonly used protocol, but one that we believe needs to be updated to reflect current knowledge:

Current (Outdated) Treatment Protocol for Children and Adults:

- Initial intramuscular (IM) or subcutaneous (SC) injections of vitamin B$_{12}$, 1,000 mcg daily or every other day for five to seven days, followed by:

- IM or SC injections of 1,000 mcg weekly for four weeks, followed by:

- Maintenance IM or SC injections of 1,000 mcg every month. This maintenance therapy may need to be lifelong.

Under the regimen outlined above, hematologic improvements typically commence within five to seven days, and the deficiency should resolve after four weeks of therapy. If the B$_{12}$ deficiency has been long-standing, and neurological manifestations are present, it can take around six months before signs of improvement appear.

In cases where neurological signs and symptoms have been present for a year or longer, or where impairment is severe, neurological damage may be permanent. Overall, neurological symptoms are completely resolved in about 50 percent of cases. The extent of improvement depends on how long the deficiency went untreated, the age of the patient, and the severity of the deficiency.

RECOMMENDED REVISION TO B_{12} DEFICIENCY TREATMENT PROTOCOL

We agree with the first two parts of the current protocol. Maintenance therapy, however, should be titrated based on a patient's response to treatment. The frequency of B_{12} injections needs to be individualized, and patients should receive hydroxocobalamin rather than cyanocobalamin (see "Which form of cobalamin is best?" below).

Some patients do well on monthly injections; however, many do better with bimonthly, trimonthly, or even weekly injections. There is no harm in giving B_{12} more frequently. Actually, it makes more sense to maintain a steady state, rather than waiting 30 days between injections in the United States, and 60 to 90 days between injections in the United Kingdom, creating periods of relative deficiency.

We recommend teaching patients, or willing family members, to administer subcutaneous injections (similar to diabetics administering insulin). This will save time for the patient and physician, as well as money for the patient. Most patients will be able to tell how long a B_{12} injection is effective and, along with their physician, can adjust the interval accordingly. The old protocol of monthly injections for all patients is simply out of date.

Lee notes in *Wintrobe's Clinical Hematology*, "The body's ability to retain the injected B_{12} is limited. If greater than 1 mg (1,000 mcg) of B_{12} is to be stored, several injections separated by at least 24 hours need to be administered, rather than a single dose." Lee also explains that some people are "short responders" whose serum

B_{12} concentrations may drop to dangerously low levels within two weeks of an injection.[5]

To illustrate the safety of more frequent B_{12} injections, let's examine the treatment of cyanide poisoning, which uses *hydroxocobalamin*. The protocol calls for 5 grams of hydroxocobalamin (5,000 times the amount of a single 1 mg [1,000 mcg] B_{12} shot) diluted in 200 mL of normal saline and infused intravenously (IV) over 15 minutes. A second dose of 5 grams may be repeated for a total dose of 10 grams in adults. The rate of the second infusion may range from 15 minutes (for patients in extremis) to two hours, as clinically indicated. In the pediatric population (0 to 18 years), the dose is 70 mg/kg of body weight, not to exceed 5 grams. Therefore, a 12-month-old child weighing 22 pounds (10 kg) would receive 700 mg or 700,000 mcg IV. This should help alleviate the fear many physicians have of giving more frequent injections. If maintenance therapy is given weekly to an adult or child, it will add up to a mere 4 mg (4,000 mcg) over the course of an entire month.

WHICH FORM OF COBALAMIN IS BEST?

It is important to note that the toxicity of vitamin B_{12} is nil, except for extremely rare allergic reactions. B_{12} is safe, water soluble, and nontoxic. However, there are several reasons why we recommend prescribing hydroxocobalamin or methylcobalamin rather than cyanocobalamin.

First, cyanocobalamin is contraindicated in patients with Leber's hereditary optic neuropathy (LHON). These patients have an inability to clear cyanide from the body properly, and their condition can be exacerbated by the administration of cyanocobalamin. Hydroxocobalamin and methylcobalamin can, of course, be used to treat LHON patients, as they do not contain the cyano-group (cyanide). In fact, there is evidence that some cases of optic neuropathy

5 G. R. Lee, "Pernicious Anemia and Other Causes of Vitamin B_{12} (Cobalamin) Deficiency," in *Wintrobe's Clinical Hematology*, 10th ed. (Baltimore: Williams & Wilkins, 1999) 941–58.

respond dramatically to hydroxocobalamin, which acts as a cyanide antagonist.

People with hepatic dysfunction may have elevated cyanide levels, and children with inborn errors of B_{12} metabolism may have a metabolic defect involving cyanide metabolism. Other forms of cobalamin are perfectly safe in these situations. Smokers, too, have elevated cyanide levels, and research shows that hydroxocobalamin injections can decrease smokers' blood cyanide levels by 59 percent; conversely, administration of cyanocobalamin could potentially raise the cyanide levels of smokers.[6]

Children and adults can be exposed to cyanide via secondhand smoke, foods that contain cyanide, or contaminated air, water, or soil. Occupational hazards also exist; for example, many people are exposed to diesel emissions, which contain a variety of toxic compounds including cyanide.

Given the greater safety and efficacy of hydroxocobalamin and methylcobalamin (both available in the United States), we agree with physician Steve Roach, who says, "I would not expect any adverse effects in most patients with either preparation [cyanocobalamin or hydroxocobalamin]. However, it seems wise to avoid a potentially harmful form of a drug when the more physiologic variety is available and is excreted at a more desirable rate."[7]

Current evidence indicates that hydroxocobalamin is superior to cyanocobalamin. Lee notes in *Wintrobe's Clinical Hematology*, "The initial retention of hydroxocobalamin is better than that of cyanocobalamin; 28 days after injection, retention still is nearly three times greater. In addition, hydroxocobalamin is more available to cells and is processed more efficiently by them."[8]

---

6 J. C. Forsyth et al., "Hydroxocobalamin as a Cyanide Antidote: Safety, Efficacy and Pharmacokinetics in Heavily Smoking Normal Volunteers," *Journal of Toxicology and Clinical Toxicology* 31, no. 2 (1993): 277–94.
7 E. S. Roach and W. T. McLean, "Neurologic Disorders of Vitamin B_{12} Deficiency," *American Family Physician* 25, no. 1 (1982): 111–15.
8 G. R. Lee, "Pernicious Anemia and Other Causes of Vitamin B_{12} (Cobalamin) Deficiency," in *Wintrobe's Clinical Hematology*, 10th ed. (Baltimore: Williams & Wilkins, 1999) 941–58.

Methylcobalamin (available at compound pharmacies) is used in the United States and other countries. It is thought to be superior to hydroxocobalamin for treating neurological disease, but there are no studies to substantiate this claim. Its greater efficacy presumably stems, at least in part, from the fact that, like hydroxocobalamin, it does not need to be decyanated. In addition, unlike either hydroxocobalamin or cyanocobalamin, it does not need to be reduced to the (+1) state (the only form that can cross the blood-brain barrier).[9] Thus, it bypasses several potentially problematic steps in B_{12} metabolism. Studies show that a small oral dose of methylcobalamin results in a greater accumulation of cobalamin in the liver than an oral dose of cyanocobalamin.

Hydroxocobalamin is easily converted to both active forms of B_{12} (*methylcobalamin* and *adenosylcobalamin*). It has been used for decades to treat inborn errors of B_{12} metabolism in children. There are no studies comparing methylcobalamin to hydroxocobalamin. In clinical practice, we see no difference in patient response, and prefer hydroxocobalamin due to its ability to be converted to *both* active forms, as well as its lower cost.

Is oral therapy as effective as injected B₁₂?

Several studies indicate that high-dose oral cyanocobalamin (1,000–2,000 mcg daily) is equivalent to cyanocobalamin injections. A recent U.S. study, for example, demonstrated that daily high-dose oral B_{12} (2,000 mcg) was as effective in producing blood and neurological responses as a standard injectable regimen in patients with B_{12} deficiency. This study strongly supports the view that oral B_{12} at doses of 2,000 mcg can replace injection therapy in

---

9 Researchers have proposed that there are approximately four steps required to convert cyanocobalamin to the active coenzyme forms (methylcobalamin and adenosylcobalamin).* Methylcobalamin is found in blood plasma, cerebrospinal fluid, and the cytosol of cells. Adenosylcobalamin predominates in cellular tissues, where it is retained in the mitochondria. If there is a defect preventing the conversion of cyanocobalamin to the active forms, it is partially or entirely unusable.

* See E. Pezacka, R. Green, and D. W. Jacobsen, "Glutathionylcobalamin as an Intermediate in the Formation of Cobalamin Coenzymes," *Biochemical and Biophysical Research Communications* 2 (1990): 443–50.

some situations. Although this was a very small study with only 33 patients, it used serum MMA and Hcy markers, demonstrating a reduction in these metabolites.[10]

However, the research on oral B_{12} is fairly sparse, and we have seen cases in which injected B_{12} resulted in far greater benefits than oral supplementation. We believe that additional research is needed to confirm the efficacy and safety of oral B_{12} for patients whose deficiencies stem from a variety of causes. Studies need to compare oral methylcobalamin to oral cyanocobalamin, and compare injectable hydroxocobalamin and methylcobalamin to oral and injectable cyanocobalamin. It is important to note that over-the-counter oral, sublingual, nasal, and transdermal B_{12} formulations are not regulated by the Food and Drug Administration. Also, remember that patients prescribed *any* form of B_{12} treatment must be monitored for efficacy, improvement or resolution of symptoms, or failure to respond.

Emmanuel Andres, M.D., notes in the *Annals of Pharmacotherapy*: "As Lane and Rojas-Fernandez demonstrated, to date only case reports or small studies have focused on oral vitamin B_{12} therapy for the treatment of cobalamin deficiencies. Thus, the ideal doses of oral cobalamin and treatment duration remain to be determined. . . . In several studies, cobalamin deficiency is not well established, be it low serum vitamin B_{12} concentrations or true cobalamin deficiency with biological or clinical features; nor is the etiology known, be it nutritional deficiency, pernicious anemia, or food-cobalamin malabsorption. To our knowledge, these limitations involve major difficulties with interpretation of the data."[11] Lane and Rojas-Fernandez concluded in their summary, "There are inadequate data at the present time to support the use of oral

10 A. M. Kuzminski et al., "Effective Treatment of Cobalamin Deficiency with Oral Cobalamin," *Blood* 92, no. 4 (1998): 1191–98.
11 E. Andrès, Comment, "Treatment of Vitamin B_{12} Deficiency Anemia: Oral versus Parenteral Therapy," *Annals of Pharmacotherapy* 36 (2002): 1268–72.

cyanocobalamin replacement in patients with severe neurological involvement."[12]

Comparing oral to injectable forms of B_{12}, Anand Sridhar, Ph.D., Wegmans School of Pharmacy, St. John Fisher College, notes: "The injectable forms are sterile preparations. Care is taken to ensure that the active ingredient (drug, vitamin, etc.) is not exposed to high stresses like heat, light, atmospheric oxygen, or acid that could affect the active ingredient's chemical nature. During their manufacture, the exposure to these stresses is kept to a minimum."

He goes on to note that, in contrast: "Oral formulations, particularly tablets, are exposed to different stresses than injectable forms. In addition to the active ingredient (drug, vitamin, etc.), a tablet contains excipients, which form the matrix in which the active ingredient resides. The process of making a tablet involves

---

FOOD FOR THOUGHT

If 1,000 mcg of oral B_{12} is equivalent to 1,000 mcg of injectable B_{12}, as some studies are suggesting, why are physicians instructing patients to take the oral, sublingual, or lozenge forms daily, while an injection is given every 30 days in the United States and every 60 to 90 days in the United Kingdom? This clearly is a problem if the oral and injectable forms are to be considered equivalent in efficacy.

As mentioned previously, we believe that B_{12} injections need to be delivered more frequently—every 7, 10, or 14 days. The protocols created more than 50 years ago to treat the hematologic signs of B_{12} deficiency (as the historic name *pernicious anemia* implies) do not reflect the needs of patients who suffer neurological or psychiatric symptoms, and fail to address patients with *MTHFR* gene mutations.

---

12 L. A. Lane and C. Rojas-Fernandez, "Treatment of Vitamin B_{12}-Deficiency Anemia: Oral versus Parenteral Therapy," *Annals of Pharmacotherapy* 36 (2002): 1268–71.

> ## B$_{12}$ GETS A BAD RAP
>
> Narcotics and other mood-altering drugs are addictive, can be abused, affect patients' judgment, increase the risk of serious falls, and make driving more dangerous. Yet doctors prescribe narcotics more freely than nontoxic, water-soluble B$_{12}$. Patients who do receive B$_{12}$ often get only one injection every month or few months, and if they tell their doctors they need more, most doctors resist and treat them like drug seekers.
>
> Why are many doctors more apt to prescribe a narcotic than B$_{12}$? Because they are poorly educated about the effects of B$_{12}$ deficiency, the safety of B$_{12}$ treatment, and the proper protocols for treating B$_{12}$-deficient patients. This dangerous knowledge gap must be addressed by the medical community.

exposing the dry powder of drug and excipients to steps like sieving (to ensure all particles are of uniform size), milling (to make smaller particles), and compacting (using a physical force to literally punch a tablet into a mold). These physical stresses are not born by the injectable form, where the B$_{12}$ powder (or crystals) are dissolved in sterile water."

He concludes: "As the nature and extent of stresses is lesser (or significantly moderated) in injectable preparations than in the tablet forms, the injectable more likely retains the vitamin in the original form. The oral form could exhibit some losses due to the vagaries of the process. This also means that you have a greater assurance of the amount (or dose) of vitamin being delivered by intramuscular injection, than by tablets. This may be one of the key reasons why injectable preparations are highly preferred over oral preparations (tablets, for example)."[13]

13 Verbal and written communication from Anand Sridhar, Ph.D., Assistant Professor of Pharmaceutical Sciences at Wegmans School of Pharmacy, St. John Fisher College.

THE NEED FOR ADDITIONAL RESEARCH

While B$_{12}$ deficiency was identified nearly a hundred years ago, we still lack basic knowledge about many aspects of the disease and its treatment. To address the B$_{12}$ deficiency epidemic effectively, we need to fill in the gaps in our understanding. There are many crucial questions researchers should explore:

- What is the real threshold for B$_{12}$ deficiency? As we have noted, the serum B$_{12}$ levels currently considered acceptable in the United States and most other countries are far too low. As a result, millions of people with "normal" test results suffer from severe symptoms and many have a true deficiency (as evidenced by concurrent MMA testing). Others will become deficient in the months to come, when their injuries could have been prevented.

- In order to diagnose patients accurately, we need to be able to test them accurately. To do this, we need to answer four questions: What is the best test or group of tests to identify B$_{12}$ deficiency? Which is superior, the urinary MMA or the serum MMA? How does the HoloTC test compare to serum B$_{12}$ and MMA? And which B$_{12}$ assay is most sensitive?

- To treat patients correctly, we need to determine the best therapy for B$_{12}$ deficiency. And to do this, we need to answer the following questions: Is oral B$_{12}$ truly an acceptable alternative to injections? Which patients can use oral or sublingual therapy, and which need injections?

- There are other treatment issues we need to explore as well. For instance, rather than following the standard archaic treatment schedule, which calls for cyanocobalamin injections every month in the United States and hydroxocobalamin injections every three months in the United Kingdom, would patients benefit more from using hydroxocobalamin injections weekly, bi-monthly, or tri-monthly?

- If clinicians prescribed injectable hydroxocobalamin as often as they do injectable methylcobalamin, would their patients show similar improvement? (We firmly believe that the answer to this and the previous question is *yes*.)

- In addition, we need to determine which forms of B_{12} are the most effective. For example: Is injectable hydroxocobalamin more effective and stable than injectable methylcobalamin?

Moreover, we need to elucidate fully the relationship between B_{12} deficiency and autism, as well as other developmental disabilities. To do this, researchers need to answer the following questions:

- How many children diagnosed with autism spectrum disorders actually suffer from an unidentified B_{12} deficiency or BABI?

- Can suboptimal or low B_{12} during fetal development and/or infancy cause mild brain injury that manifests as high-functioning autism?

- Can overt B_{12} deficiency in fetal development and/or infancy cause moderate- to low-functioning autism?

- What effect would universal screening of children with developmental delay for B_{12} deficiency have on the identification of children who might otherwise be diagnosed with "incurable" autism?

- Would screening women for B_{12} deficiency during pregnancy and breastfeeding (using urinary MMA) significantly reduce the rates of autism and developmental delay?

- Would high-dose oral/sublingual biologically active B_{12} (1,000 mcg daily) taken by women before conception, during pregnancy, and during breastfeeding reduce the rising rates of autism spectrum disorders?

- Should pregnant women also receive monthly hydroxocobalamin shots during their prenatal visits?

- Should the lower-end normal value for serum B$_{12}$ in infants and young children be raised to 1,000 pg/mL to promote neurological health?

- Should the medical community and government agencies involved in public health care create new guidelines that promote early identification of B$_{12}$ deficiency in infants by testing them at the ages of 6 and 12 months using the noninvasive urine MMA assay?

- Are some cases of cerebral palsy caused by unknown B$_{12}$ deficiency that injures the brain during fetal growth and development? (See Megan's story in Chapter 5.)

- How many women are receiving nitrous oxide during pregnancy and/or during delivery?

- How many children are receiving nitrous oxide?

- Are carriers of the *MTHFR* gene mutation more susceptible to B$_{12}$ deficiency, BABI, and SCD when other accompanying insults are present (e.g., a vegan/vegetarian diet, nitrous oxide exposure, or proton-pump inhibitor use)?

- How much money is spent on lengthy hospitalization (neonatal intensive care units) of newborns because of low birth weight (LBW) caused by B$_{12}$ deficiency, as well as the complications that arise from LBW and B$_{12}$ deficiency?

- How much money is spent on hospitalization and diagnostic work-ups of critically ill children with neurological and hematologic complications of chronic B$_{12}$ deficiency?

- How much money is spent on costly infertility treatments and doctors not investigating if B$_{12}$ deficiency or a genetic mutation is involved?

Currently, most medical professionals are unaware of the neuropsychiatric manifestations of B$_{12}$ deficiency and the role that this deficiency plays in developmental disorders (and, in particular, autism). The minority of doctors who *are* aware of B$_{12}$'s role in

---

SHOULD ALL NEWBORNS RECEIVE INJECTABLE B$_{12}$?

Currently, the American Academy of Pediatrics recommends giving vitamin K to all newborns as a single, intramuscular injection. This is because it is believed to be the most effective and efficient way of protecting babies from vitamin K deficiency bleeding, and more easily absorbed than oral drops. While vitamin K deficiency is rare (incidence of 0.25 percent to 1.7 percent), it has been standard practice since 1961 to give this vitamin as a preventative measure to all infants whether or not risk factors are present.

Unlike vitamin K deficiency, B$_{12}$ deficiency is not rare. And B$_{12}$ deficiency, like vitamin K deficiency, seriously endangers infants. Therefore, should health-care systems consider giving hydroxocobalamin injections to all newborns (as they do vitamin K) to prevent the devastating neurological complications of low B$_{12}$?

Taking it one step further, should hydroxocobalamin injections be given monthly during pregnancy and breastfeeding as a preventative measure? These injections are cheap, cost-effective, and nontoxic, and would provide powerful protection for pregnant women and their unborn children.

---

autism typically prescribe frequent high-dose injections of methyl-B$_{12}$ to autistic children without first performing tests to determine their true B$_{12}$ status. These physicians, while well intentioned, are actually preventing us from obtaining crucial information about the role of B$_{12}$ deficiency in autism. The same is true of parents who treat children on the autism spectrum with B$_{12}$ without first having these children tested.

It is imperative that we begin to investigate, document, and report the true incidence of cobalamin deficiency in children (particular those with symptoms of autism or developmental disability), in women of childbearing age, and in patients with mental illness. When we do this, we will be able to accurately determine the magnitude of this problem and take steps to address it.

151

A RISK-BENEFIT ANALYSIS OF B$_{12}$ DEFICIENCY DIAGNOSIS AND TREATMENT

In medicine, we constantly weigh the risks and benefits of tests and treatments. For example, CT scans can provide us with crucial diagnostic information, but they also expose our patients to potentially dangerous radiation. And heart surgery may cure a patient, but it can also be fatal.

When it comes to risks and benefits, however, B$_{12}$ deficiency is in a category all its own. That's because there are *no* risks involved in diagnosing the problem (which requires only some simple lab tests) or in treating it. Both diagnosis and treatment are inexpensive, as we'll show in the next chapter. And the benefits are incalculable. We personally know scores of B$_{12}$-deficient patients who were spared from permanent disability or even death by a doctor's intervention.

In short, while many medical decisions are agonizing, this one is simple. Be aggressive in testing and treating your patients. It may take you a few extra minutes of time, and add a few hundred dollars to a patient's bill, but that's a very small price to pay for saving a life.

13

Dollars and Sense: The Cost Effectiveness of Screening and Treating Patients for B₁₂ Deficiency

Health-care costs are astronomical and continue to rise every year. As medical professionals, we understand that we have a serious responsibility to consider these costs when we diagnose and treat patients. However, one of the worst mistakes that the medical community can make is to be "penny wise and pound foolish." When we cut corners by failing to diagnose and treat our patients correctly, we don't just cause them injury or pain. In addition, we harm them—and society—financially.

One of the clearest examples of this is B_{12} deficiency. Of course, money is probably your lowest priority if you're worried about your own health or the health of your child. But we think it's important for medical consumers to understand why the medical community's rampant failure to diagnose this problem costs patients, insurers, and society dearly.

In addition to direct clinical costs related to B_{12}-associated conditions and the inevitable waste of health-care dollars that results from misdiagnosis, it's important to consider as well the potentially catastrophic financial burdens borne by patients and their families when chronic illness and disability leads to loss of income or livelihood.

ONE PATIENT'S STORY

George Rossetti, a career medical writer/editor, was court-declared disabled as of December 2010, when symptoms of advanced subacute combined degeneration (SCD) at last rendered him unemployable. (George's struggles with B$_{12}$ deficiency are described in the foreword he contributed to this book.) His medical history is complex, and ongoing management, monitoring, and treatment are very expensive.

Currently, George receives Medicare benefits, has decent secondary health insurance through his wife Donna's policy, and is eligible for Veterans Administration (VA) benefits due to service-related disability. For now, at least, out-of-pocket costs for health care are manageable, and he's thankful for that. But the realities of George's sudden unemployment proved at least as stressful and frightening as his symptoms.

"In addition to the day-to-day struggles of living with chronic illness and disability," George wrote, "another life-altering consequence of my missed diagnosis that hit us very hard, of course, was a sudden and dramatic loss of income. I went from earning a comfortable six-figure salary to drawing subsistence-level SSDI [Social Security Disability Insurance]." As a result of this staggering loss of income, George and Donna had to make substantial life-style adjustments and reconsider long-held plans for their future and retirement.

Furthermore, acquiring SSDI benefits is hardly a sure thing. George recalls, "One reason the administrative law judge quickly found in my favor for SSDI benefits was credibility. It made absolutely no sense for a man at my income level, with my resume, robust employment history, professional achievements, and future prospects to go to so much trouble, at age 55, to throw it all away in exchange for what amounts to a very modest pension. So, in addition to the persuasive mountain of medical evidence before the judge, he reasoned that "only a fool would willingly walk away from the stability and security I once had…unless he had no choice."

Despite all the hard clinical evidence from physicians and George's credibility, a disengaged or ill-tempered judge could easily have denied benefits, forcing an exhaustive, time-consuming appeal. "Applying for SSDI is an unpleasant, frustrating, and at times a humiliating process. People who truly deserve benefits are routinely denied, while favorable decisions are frequently handed down to dishonest able-bodied people," George added.

Despite all, George feels relatively lucky, under the circumstances. "Barring further setbacks, Donna and I will get by," he feels. "It's just the two of us, and our combined incomes—though drastically reduced—should suffice for our needs. Ours is an unfortunate case, but not as tragic as it might have been. I can't imagine how we would survive this if we had children and all the incumbent responsibilities."

If only doctors were up to date on B_{12} deficiency, George and countless others wouldn't have to suffer life-long disability and financial hardship. George does have the medical documentation to pursue a malpractice case, but has chosen not to do so.

THE SMALL PRICE OF SCREENING VERSUS THE HIGH COST OF FAILING TO SCREEN

When doctors fail to diagnose B_{12} deficiency, the financial cost to their patients can be staggering. These patients make appointment after appointment with specialists, undergo dozens of expensive and often unnecessary tests, and receive prescriptions for costly medications that provide no benefit. Often, they wind up in the emergency room or need to be hospitalized.

As children's development regresses and their neurological symptoms are misdiagnosed as autism, these children will need language, speech, occupational, and physical therapies. Likewise, as adults' neurological symptoms grow worse, many need physical therapy, suffer traumatic injuries from falls, or need to use scooters or other mobility aids because they are no longer able to walk. As they become more and more anemic, patients often need costly blood transfusions or erythropoietin treatment. If their deficiency affects them mentally, patients may spend thousands of dollars on psychiatric care and medications or even need psychiatric hospitalization. Many elderly patients develop dementia as a result of undiagnosed or late-diagnosed B$_{12}$ deficiency and require 24-hour supervision or nursing home care.

As George's story earlier illustrated, people with chronic misdiagnosed B$_{12}$ deficiency frequently end up on disability after suffering profoundly debilitating neurological or cognitive damage. Many dip into their life savings, becoming bankrupt or even homeless.

Clearly, in addition to placing lives in jeopardy, doctors who miss a diagnosis of B$_{12}$ deficiency cause patients and society tremendous financial harm. In addition, these doctors are putting themselves at risk for malpractice suits if other medical professionals correctly diagnose their patients, documenting deficiency with appropriate tests, and revealing the original doctors' negligence.

So why do medical professionals rarely screen patients for this common medical problem? Is it because B$_{12}$ screening is expensive? The answer to this question is a resounding *no*. Table 13.1 compares B$_{12}$ screening to other diagnostic tests.

TABLE 13.1: COSTS OF B$_{12}$ TESTING VS. OTHER DIAGNOSTIC BLOOD TESTS

Lab Tests for B$_{12}$ Deficiency	Cost
Vitamin B$_{12}$	$50
Urinary MMA	$150
Serum MMA	$150
HoloTC (Active B$_{12}$)	$118
Homocysteine	$147

Other Commonly Ordered Blood Tests	Cost
Complete blood cell (CBC) count w/diff	$43
Serum iron	$48
Ferritin	$101
Transferrin	$59
TSH	$119
T-4 (free)	$162
BNP	$257
Lipid profile	$90
Hemoglobin A1C	$62
Blood glucose	$23
Vitamin D, 25-hydroxy	$124

There is a misconception that B_{12} screening is not cost effective compared to other screening tests; however, this is untrue. The 25-hydroxy vitamin D test costs $124, yet physicians routinely order it. Ruling out iron deficiency costs over $200, screening for hypothyroidism costs $281, and screening for diabetes costs $81. Routine cholesterol testing costs $90, and physicians often order the B-type natriuretic peptide (BNP) test, at a cost of $257, to determine the presence and/or severity of heart failure. By comparison, a serum B_{12} test costs an average of $50, and the MMA tests cost $150.

Now, let's examine the cost of B_{12} testing for women who are pregnant or breastfeeding. B_{12} and urinary MMA testing—which are relatively inexpensive, as you've seen—are crucial during these times. In addition, *MTHFR* genotyping needs to be considered for women who are pregnant or trying to get pregnant, to ascertain if they need to be placed on special prenatal vitamins (active B_{12}, B_9, and B_6). This test costs $182 and may be a lifesaver for many women and their children.

To place the cost of B_{12} testing in perspective, Table 13.2 lists the costs of prenatal tests routinely ordered for women in the first trimester.

TABLE 13.2: STANDARD TESTS DURING THE FIRST TRIMESTER OF PREGNANCY

Lab Tests for B_{12} Deficiency	Cost
Rubella immunity	$80
Hepatitis B	$85
HIV I/II	$85
Syphilis	$29
Blood type, Rh (rhesus) factor	$27
Antibody screen	$36
Ultrasound pregnancy complete <14 weeks	$530–$811

Every pregnant woman in the United States is tested for syphilis, HIV, and hepatitus, even if they are not at risk. Yet our health-care system fails to test for maternal B_{12} deficiency, or *MTHFR* genotyping, which—like these other diseases—can cause a child or a mother to suffer serious intellectual and neurological disabilities, or can even be fatal.

From a financial perspective, it is foolish to skimp on B_{12} testing for pregnant or breastfeeding women or their infants (who, in our opinion, should have a urinary MMA test performed at 6 and 12 months of age). A failure to diagnose B_{12} deficiency in pregnant or breastfeeding women or their children leads to massive costs in other areas, including hospitalization in neonatal units and pediatric intensive care units. In older patients, these costs also include hospitalization and rehabilitation care for patients whose symptoms continue to go misdiagnosed and worsen. B_{12} deficiency frequently causes fall-related trauma, and patients who present with injuries caused by falls require X-rays or CT scans. A CT of the brain without contrast costs on average $987, and a hip and femur X-ray costs $669. Table 13.3 shows the cost of room rates for hospitalization. This table does not include physician fees, treatment fees, equipment, supplies, or medications.

TABLE 13.3: COSTS OF HOSPITALIZATION (2014)

Description	Charges per Day
Emergency room visit (level 4)	$916
Room and board, psychiatric facility	$768
Room and board, semiprivate bed	$1,004
Room and board, telemetry bed	$1,530
Room and board for ICU medical or ICU surgical bed	$3,304
Room and board, rehabilitation facility bed	$500
Long-term care (nursing home)	$220/day $6,700/month $80,400/year

To analyze the costs of a missed B_{12}-deficiency diagnosis from another perspective, let's explore five different consequences of B_{12} deficiency.

1. MENTAL ILLNESS

As we discussed in Chapter 9, undiagnosed B_{12} deficiency can cause depression as well as a wide range of other mental symptoms ranging from paranoia to hallucinations. Doctors often fail to screen patients with these symptoms for B_{12} deficiency, choosing instead to prescribe antidepressants and other psychotropic drugs. In doing this, they condemn many B_{12}-deficient patients to a lifetime of mental illness, and they waste millions of health-care dollars as well.

For example, we told the story of a woman who developed bipolar disorder as a result of B$_{12}$ deficiency. This woman was prescribed thousands of dollars' worth of psychotropic drugs and then required emergency room treatment and hospitalization—costing many more thousands of dollars—when she became suicidal.

While the cost of such mistakes in human terms is incalculable, we can determine some of the financial costs. Table 13.4 lists the costs of some commonly prescribed antidepressant and psychiatric medications—as well as the annual cost of self-administered hydroxocobalamin (B$_{12}$) shots.

DEPRESSION, OR B$_{12}$ DEFICIENCY?

An 18-year-old woman came to our emergency department (ED) after experiencing suicidal thoughts. She'd already been treated by a physician and prescribed psychiatric medications. The doctor instructed the teen's mother to bring her to the ED for medical clearance and psychiatric hospitalization.

The physician in the ED included B$_{12}$ testing in the teen's medical clearance, and she proved to have a severe B$_{12}$ deficiency (B$_{12}$ less than 160 pg/mL). Injectable B$_{12}$ treatment was begun in the ED, and the ED physician ordered daily B$_{12}$ injections during the woman's psychiatric admission.

The ED physician explained to both the patient and her mom that an underlying medical condition was causing or at least greatly contributing to her severe depression, and that this condition was treatable. This was very good news for both the patient and her mother. And from a financial perspective, this doctor's excellent diagnostic work undoubtedly saved this family—as well as the health care system—many thousands of dollars.

TABLE 13.4: COSTS OF PROPRIETARY AND GENERIC ANTIDEPRESSANT AND PSYCHIATRIC MEDICATIONS VERSUS HYDROXOCOBALAMIN

Medication*	Dose	Cost Per Month	Cost per Year
Abilify	2 mg daily	$890	$10,680
aripiprazole	Cost not available at press time		
Celexa	10 mg daily	$172	$2,064
citalopram		*$29*	*$348*
Cymbalta	30 mg daily	$252	$3,024
duloxetine		*$221*	*$2,652*
Lexapro	10 mg daily	$196	$2,352
escitalopram		*$101*	*$1,212*
Prozac	10 mg daily	$254	$3,048
fluoxetine		*$19*	*$230*
Risperdal	4 mg once daily	$680	$8,157
risperidone		*$58*	*$701*
Zoloft	50 mg daily	$182	$2,184
sertraline		*$20*	*$240*
Hydroxocobalamin, injectable (30 mL vial)	1,000 mcg IM bi-monthly or 500 mcg SC weekly (this also includes the loading dose of six initial daily injections).	$3	$36

*Proprietary names and costs of medications appear in regular font; generic names and comparative costs appear in italics.

2. NEUROLOGICAL PROBLEMS

Many children, teens, and adults with B_{12} deficiency develop neurological symptoms. For instance, they may experience vision problems, lose their ability to walk, or develop "pins and needles" sensations in their arms and legs. Doctors typically order dozens of tests for patients experiencing these symptoms, and prescribe a multitude of medications, without ever considering testing for B$_{12}$ deficiency.

Often, teenagers and young and middle-aged adults with B$_{12}$ deficiency receive a misdiagnosis of multiple sclerosis (MS) and are treated with medications for MS. That's because MS and B$_{12}$ deficiency are both demyelinating disorders and share the same symptoms. Additionally, MS and pernicious anemia are both autoimmune disorders.

Tables 13.5, 13.6, and 13.7 show a sampling of the tests doctors typically order and the medications they typically prescribe for patients with neurological symptoms, such as multiple sclerosis, along with their costs.

TABLE 13.5: COSTS OF NEUROLOGICAL TESTS

Test	Cost
CT brain without contrast	$987
CT brain with contrast	$1,196
MRI brain without contrast	$1,250
MRI brain with and without contrast	$1,950
MRI C-spine, T-spine, LS-spine without contrast	$1,250 (each area) or $3,750 for entire spine
MRI C-spine, T-spine, LS-spine with contrast	$1,950 (each area) or $5,850 for entire spine
EMG/NCV	$150–$500 per limb All limbs $600–$2,000
EEG (awake and drowsy)	$438
EEG extended greater than 1 hour	$1,159
Acetylcholine receptor	$145
Muscle weakness autoimmune reflexive panel (for myasthenia gravis)	$1,800–$2,200
Lumbar puncture (diagnostic) for MS	$234
Lyme antibody	$137
Lyme-confirmed Western Blot Test	$83

TABLE 13.6: COSTS OF PROPRIETARY AND GENERIC NEUROLOGICAL MEDICATIONS

Medication*	Dose	Cost per Month	Cost per Year
Ativan	1 mg once daily	$243.70	$2,924
lorazepam		*$15.99*	*$191*
Lyrica	50 mg once daily	$157.93	$1,895
pregabalin	Cost not available at press time		
Mysoline	25 mg twice daily	$152.99	$1,835
primidone		*$15.39*	*$185*
Neurontin	300 mg three times daily	$272.67	$3,272
gabapentin		*$59.69*	*$716*
Zanaflex	2 mg three times daily	$269.99	$3,239
tizanidine		*$217.99*	*$2,615*

*Proprietary names and costs of medications appear in regular font; generic names and comparative costs appear in italics.

TABLE 13.7: COSTS OF MEDICATIONS PRESCRIBED FOR MULTIPLE SCLEROSIS

Medication	Dose	Cost per Month	Cost per Year
Avonex	30 mg subcutaneously weekly	$5,454	$65,448
Betaseron (*interferon beta 1b*)	0.3 mg subcutaneously every other day	$5,654	$67,854
Copaxone	20 mg subcutaneously daily	$6,682	$80,191
Extavia	0.3 mg subcutaneously every other day	$5,777	$69,332
Gilenya	0.5 mg orally every day	$6,886	$82,635

3. B$_{12}$-deficiency acquired brain injury (BABI)

Currently, one in every 68 children is diagnosed as autistic. As we noted in Chapter 8, B$_{12}$ deficiency in infants and children causes developmental delay and can easily be mistaken for autism. It is unknown how many children labeled as autistic have B$_{12}$-deficiency Acquired Brain Injury (BABI), but our guess is that the number is high.

Identifying such children *before* they suffer brain injury would prevent many tragedies, and it would reap huge savings in healthcare dollars. Michael Ganz, Assistant Professor of Society, Human Development, and Health at Harvard School of Public Health, puts the lifetime cost of caring for one autistic child at approximately $3.2 million.[1] But Ganz believes this is likely an underestimate, because it includes only medical costs, such as visits to doctors' offices, medications, and therapies; and nonmedical costs, such as adult care, childcare, and special education; and does not include costs due to lost parental income and lost income for people with autism.

The cost of lifelong care for a patient with BABI is similar to the cost of care for an individual with autism. Table 13.8 highlights the costs of occupational and speech therapy, as well as a typical autism program.

Table 13.8: Therapies/Programs for Children with Autism

Therapy	Initial Evaluation	Cost per Session	Cost per Week	Cost per Month	Cost per Year
Speech and Language	$255	$149 (45 minutes)	$298 (2 x per week)	$1,192	$14,304
Occupational	$185	$168 (30 minutes)	$336 (2 x per week)	$1,344	$16,128
Physical	$185	$168 (30 minutes)	$336 (2 x per week)	$1,344	$16,128
Autism Program*			$750	$3,000**	$36,000
All 4 therapies	Not included in total cost				$82,560

* **Applied Behavior Analysis (3 hours per day, 15 hours per week, Monday–Friday, 20 days per month)**
** **20 (3 hour) sessions in a 4-week period**

1 M. L. Ganz, "The Lifetime Distribution of the Incremental Societal Costs of Autism," *Archives of Pediatric and Adolescent Medicine* 161, no. 4 (2007): 343–49.

Table 13.9 outlines common medications used to treat children on the autism spectrum (as well as children with ADD and/or ADHD).

Table 13.9: Proprietary and Generic Medications Commonly Prescribed for Children with Autism

Medication*	Dose & Frequency	Cost per Month	Cost per Year
Adderall	20 mg once daily	$263.75	$3,165
dextroamphetamine		*$219.12*	*$2,629*
Concerta	36 mg once daily	$296.09	$3,229
methylphenidate		*$195.01*	*$2,340*
Focalin XR	30 mg once daily	$228.74	$3,464
dexmethylphenidate		*$201.76*	*$2,421*
Intuniv	2 mg once daily	$299.64	$3,595
guanfacine	*Cost not available at press time*		
Klonopin	1 mg twice daily	$166.65	$1,999
clonazepam		*$25.64*	*$307*
Risperdal	2 mg once daily	$426.40	$5,112
risperidone		*$50*	*$600*
Ritalin	20 mg once daily	$53.70	$644
methylphenidate		*$52.84*	*$634*
Seroquel	50 mg twice daily	$435.31	$5,223
quetiapine		*$97.73*	*$1,172*
Strattera	40 mg once daily	$302.65	$3,631
no generic			
Vivance XR	50 mg once daily	$246.36	$2,956
no generic			
Wellbutrin XL	150 mg once daily	$445.39	$5,344
bupropion		*$48.72*	*$584*
Zyprexa	10 mg once daily	$635.96	$7,631
olanzapine		*$149.85*	*$1,798*

*Proprietary names and costs of medications appear in regular font; generic names and comparative costs appear in italics.

Autism is largely considered an incurable disorder. Low B$_{12}$, by contrast, is simple to diagnose, and early treatment often leads to a complete cure. However, when low B$_{12}$ turns into B$_{12}$ deficiency and diagnosis is delayed, children (as well as adults) may improve to some degree, but typically will have a lifelong neurological injury or intellectual disability. Viewed from a financial perspective, each early diagnosis of pediatric B$_{12}$ deficiency that would otherwise become BABI can save society of millions of dollars. That's a huge return on an investment of only a few hundred dollars' worth of lab tests.

Consider the following: The amount of money spent by the government, insurance companies, and taxpayers to care for *one* BABI child could have been used to screen 16,000 at-risk or symptomatic children. Remember, studies show that 3 percent of children (1 in 33) under the age of 4 are B$_{12}$-deficient,[2] and an unknown percentage—15 percent, if the number is similar to that for adults—are low in B$_{12}$. Low B$_{12}$ (200–300 pg/mL) is often shown to be a true B$_{12}$ deficiency when the MMA test is used.

4. ANEMIA

Infants and young children can become very anemic and develop other blood count abnormalities as a result of B$_{12}$ deficiency. When this happens, doctors often end up performing a bone marrow biopsy to rule out leukemia. In addition, these children frequently receive blood transfusions. Both biopsies and transfusions are costly and can lead to complications. These interventions can be avoided with early B$_{12}$-deficiency screening and diagnosis.

In the emergency department, we see adult patients whose anemia is so severe as a result of B$_{12}$ deficiency that they too require blood transfusions. Many patients with undiagnosed B$_{12}$ deficiency have endoscopies and colonoscopies performed because their doctors are searching for bleeding to explain their severe anemia. These procedures are costly; in 2014 the average cost of a colo-

2 L. H. Allen, "How Common Is Vitamin B-12 Deficiency?" *American Journal of Clinical Nutrition* 89, no. 2 (2009): 693S–696S.

noscopy was $2,750 and an esophagogastroduodenoscopy (EGD) was $1,750. Moreover, they are not without risk, exposing patients to anesthesia as well as the possibility of accidental perforation or exposure to blood-borne diseases. After all of this testing, when no cause for the anemia is found, these patients are sent home, only to return months later to repeat the process, all because B_{12} deficiency was not contemplated.

Patients with chronic anemia due to cancer or renal failure often receive erythropoietin (Procrit or Epogen) to improve their anemia. In these cases as well, physicians routinely screen for iron deficiency but typically do not screen for B_{12} deficiency. Yet clearly, it is not cost effective to place a patient on Procrit, which costs approximately $5,866 for eight weeks of treatment, without ruling out low B_{12} as a cause of the anemia.

5. Gastric bypass surgery (GBS)

Each year, more than 140,000 Americans undergo GBS for weight loss. Doctors recommend GBS for obese patients because they believe it will prevent death or disability. And in many cases, it does. But in many other cases, patients wind up in greater danger than before their surgeries. We have seen countless GBS patients arrive at the emergency department with severe anemia, fall-related trauma, or mental status changes because their health-care providers failed to understand that gastric bypass surgery will cause severe B_{12} deficiency over time unless patients receive proper lifelong B_{12} supplementation.

For example, one patient came to our ER because she was experiencing psychological and neurological symptoms. Her primary care doctor sent her to the ER to rule out a transient ischemic attack (mini-stroke), even though her symptoms were bilateral, while stroke symptoms occur on only one side of the body. As it turned out, she had severe B_{12} deficiency stemming from her GBS four years earlier. Her hospital admission and the array of tests she received before getting her B_{12}-deficiency diagnosis cost more than $18,000 (cost in 2009 dollars).

SAVING BILLIONS OF DOLLARS—BY SPENDING PENNIES PER PATIENT PER DAY

As you can see from the numbers in this chapter, undiagnosed B$_{12}$ deficiency costs society billions of dollars annually. Now, let's look at the other side of the coin: How much does it cost to treat B$_{12}$ deficiency correctly? The answer, astonishingly, is less than 12 cents per person per day.

If you're curious, here's the math. In 2014, a 30 mL vial of injectable B$_{12}$ (hydroxocobalamin 1,000 mcg/mL) costs on average between \$32 and \$41. Dividing \$32 and \$41 by 365 yields a daily cost of 9 cents and 11 cents, respectively. This cost includes the initial series of injections followed by maintenance therapy. A 30 mL vial of B$_{12}$ contains enough for a patient to receive six initial injections (1,000 mcg) every day or every other day, leaving a sufficient amount for bi-monthly 1,000 mcg injections over the next 12 months. Methyl-B$_{12}$ lozenges are slightly more expensive, costing around 12 to 38 cents per day depending on the strength. That's still quite a bargain, though as we've noted, more research needs to be done on the efficacy of oral B$_{12}$ treatment.

Tables 13.10 and 13.11 list the monthly and yearly costs of different prescription and nonprescription forms of B$_{12}$.

Table 13.10: Monthly and Yearly Costs of Different Forms of B_{12}

Prescription (Rx) B_{12} and nonprescription B_{12}	Cost per Month	Cost per Year
Folgard cyanocobalamin 115 mcg folic acid 800 mcg vitamin B_6 10 mg	$23.37	$280
Folgard RX (Rx) Cyanocobalamin 1,000 mcg Folic acid 2.2 mg Vitamin B_6 25mg	$25.68 $19.92 generic	$308 $239 generic
Metanx (Rx) Methylcobalamin 2 mg L-methylfolate 3 mg Pyridoxal 5'-phosphate 35 mg No generic	$74.54	$894
Cerefolin (Rx) Methylcobalamin 2 mg L-methylfolate 5.6 mg N-acetylcysteine 600 mg No generic	$129.39	$1,552
Nascobal nasal spray (Rx) Cyanocobalamin 500 mcg/spray (1.3 mL) 4 doses prescribed weekly 1-month supply	$471.99	$5,663
Methyl-B_{12} lozenges 1,000 mcg daily (non-Rx) OTC (100 for $12.00)	$3.60	$43
Methyl-B_{12} lozenges 5,000 mcg daily (non-Rx) OTC (2 leading brands)	$6.50–$11.45	$78–$137
B_{12} transdermal patch 1,000 mcg (4 patches) applied once weekly (efficacy not studied)	$40	$480

TABLE 13.11: MONTHLY AND YEARLY COST OF INJECTABLE B₁₂

Medication	Qty.	Dispensed	Cost per Month	Cost per Year
Cyanocobalamin (injectable) 1,000 mcg/mL = 1 mg/mL monthly	1 mL	1 vial = 1mL 1 injection	$8.78	$105
Cyanocobalamin (injectable) 1 mg/mL bi-monthly	1 mL	2 vials = 2 mL 2 injections	$14.86	$178
Hydroxocobalamin (injectable) 1 mg/mL bi-monthly + initial 6 injections 1 mg = 1,000 mcg Manufactured by Hikma Farmaceutica (Portugal) Distributed by Watson Pharma, Inc. USA NDC 0591-2888-30 Not made by compounding pharmacy	30 mL	30 mL multi-dose vial 30 injections	$2.66– $3.42	$32– $41
Methylcobalamin (injectable) 25 mg/mL yields 25 doses 0.04 mL x 25 doses = 1 mL 0.04 mL = 1,000 mcg or 1 mg of methyl-B₁₂ 0.04 mL is 4 units on insulin syringe. Expires in 30 days. Costs more because it is made by a compounding pharmacy.	1 mL yields 25 doses		$25	$300
Methylcobalamin (injectable) prefilled syringe 1 mg or 1,000 mcg/syringe Available in 0.04 and 0.08 mL	$4.50 per syringe	8, twice weekly 4, once weekly 2, bi-monthly	$36 $18 $9	$432 $216 $108

The bottom line: saving lives and saving money

At a time when cost containment is crucial for the medical community, one of the simplest and most effective cost-cutting steps that medical professionals can take is to address the B_{12} deficiency epidemic. Failing to do this costs society billions of dollars annually for medical tests and treatments, nursing home or residential care, and disability payments. By comparison, the solution to this problem—testing for B_{12} deficiency and providing effective treatment for those who need it—costs next to nothing. The necessary tests add up to only a few hundred dollars per person, and we can provide treatment for around a dime a day.

So why does B_{12} deficiency continue to destroy so many lives and cost society so many billions of dollars? The answer is simple: Both consumers and medical providers are unaware of the problem. To end the epidemic of B_{12} deficiency, we must educate medical professionals, the public, the media, and government officials about the need for B_{12} testing and treatment, as well as preventing deficiency in the first place. In the next chapter, we lay out an effective plan for accomplishing this crucial goal.

14

A Call for a United Effort

In this book, we have exposed a major breakdown in the medical systems in America and around the world. An epidemic of B_{12} deficiency is raging, invisible to the public, and virtually undetected by medical professionals. A safe, simple, and inexpensive treatment exists, but only a minority of sufferers ever receive this, or even an accurate diagnosis. As a result, millions of people are affected by this disorder, many are injured, and some even lose their lives.

Clearly, action is needed to combat this epidemic. All of us involved in health care must stand up for the patients who count on us. This includes not only physicians, nurses, and other direct-care providers, but all others in a position to take positive action. For example:

- Teachers and other professionals treating children with developmental disabilities must understand the role that B_{12} deficiency can play in these disorders, and they must advocate for B_{12} screening.

- Mental health professionals and psychiatric facilities must insist on B_{12} screening as part of their basic workup for all patients, including those with postpartum depression or postpartum psychosis.

- Federal, state, and local agencies and publicly funded health-care systems (such as Britain's NHS) that provide medical screenings and other health-care services for children, pregnant or nursing women, and the elderly need to make proper B_{12} screening part of their routine services.

- Nursing home and assisted living administrators must include B_{12} testing for all of their residents and provide treatment for those in the *gray zone*. (See chapter 11).

- Medical insurers and government agencies involved in health care must promote B_{12} awareness as a means of dramatically reducing health-care expenses.

- Nurse case managers and clinical social workers must become aware of the problem of B_{12} deficiency and the role it plays in causing low birth weight, developmental delays, mental illness, intellectual and cognitive disabilities, physical disabilities, fall-related trauma, reduced independence, and crowding of our emergency department, psychiatric, and long-term care facilities.

Consumers, too, must accept the responsibility for protecting their own health. To do this, they must insist on proper diagnosis and treatment if they are at risk or develop symptoms consistent with B_{12} deficiency. In addition, they must protect their loved ones—especially their children and their aging parents or grandparents—by serving as their advocates. Each of us must play our part in stopping the B_{12} epidemic—but to be truly effective, this effort must reach the highest levels.

Thus, we call on the Surgeon General of the United States, officials who head the National Health Service (NHS) of the United Kingdom, and other countries' health-care leaders to implement an immediate *Call for Action* to combat B_{12} deficiency. This easily diagnosed condition can be treated effectively for a few dollars per month per patient, or literally 12 cents per day. Conversely, left undiagnosed, it costs the world's health-care systems billions of dollars each year. We believe this is among the most crucial issues for leading health-care authorities to address.

Because B_{12} deficiency knows no borders, a new protocol and standard-of-care change must be implemented by the global medical community. In particular, B_{12} deficiency must be included on the list of *Never Events* in the United States and United Kingdom and in similar preventative initiatives throughout the world.

Never Events are serious, largely preventable patient safety incidents that should never occur once appropriate preventative measures have been implemented. For instance, in the United States, one Never Event is a death or serious disability associated with a fall suffered by a patient while in a health-care facility. It is ironic that B_{12} deficiency commonly causes falls in people of any age, yet we fail to include B_{12} deficiency as a Never Event in governmental and health-care environments.

And consider another Never Event in the United States—death or serious disability associated with failure to identify and treat hyperbilirubinemia in newborns. We fully agree that this needs to be a Never Event. But is death or serious disability acceptable in infants or children if it stems from a failure to identify and treat vitamin B_{12} deficiency? And is a death or serious disability acceptable when it stems from a failure to identify and treat B_{12} deficiency in pregnant and breastfeeding women?

> Vitamin B_{12} deficiency is one of the most preventable and most treatable of all medical scourges—but only if we choose to act.

Clearly, B_{12} deficiency should be at the top of any Never Event list in any country. There is no excuse—ever—for patients to suffer from a life-threatening problem that is this simple to identify and treat. Remember, delayed diagnosis or treatment causes poor neurological outcomes, including brain atrophy, subacute combined degeneration (SCD) and B_{12}-deficiency Acquired Brain Injury (BABI).

175

LENNON'S STORY: WHY B₁₂ DEFICIENCY NEEDS TO BE A NEVER EVENT

In Chapter 8, we talked about Lennon Groover, who has a lifelong neurological injury due to his doctors' failure to diagnose his B₁₂ deficiency. In reality, however, Lennon was victimized twice; first by his doctors, and second by the legal system. And making B₁₂ deficiency a Never Event can prevent this from happening to children like him.

Lennon, a beautiful baby boy, began to fall behind developmentally at 9 months of age. His head stopped growing, and his weight and growth flatlined. When Lennon was 11 months old, his pediatrician diagnosed anemia and started him on iron. As the months passed, he continued to experience developmental delay. His language, speech, socialization, mobility, and eating were all regressing.

Lennon's parents, Melinda and Greg, were extremely concerned and took Lennon to their pediatrician regularly. The doctor assured them that Lennon's weakness and developmental delays were due to his previous iron deficiency anemia. He also assured them that Lennon's development was along the lines of some of his other patients, and that there was no need to worry.

At 15 months, Lennon was taken off the iron because the pediatrician told the parents his anemia had resolved. At 21 months, the pediatrician placed Lennon on a nutritional supplement called Juice Plus, and diagnosed him with anemia and failure to thrive. When Lennon continued to decline developmentally, he was referred to a pediatric neurologist who specialized in developmental delay. A detailed assessment, a brain MRI, and an array of laboratory studies were performed, including testing for eleven enzyme defects. The pediatric neurologist told Melinda and Greg that she was "100 percent sure" Lennon had a form of a rare genetic disorder called mucopolysaccharide disease.

The neurologist also referred Lennon to a pediatric endocrinologist "to evaluate him for pituitary insufficiency and for nutritional issues regarding him having been breastfed by a vegetarian mother." At 23 months of age, Lennon saw the endocrinologist, who had nothing else to add to the pediatric neurologist's diagnosis but said to follow up with her again in six months.

Lennon was now 24 months old and growing weaker. He was approaching death, but not from some incurable disease. Melinda and Greg trusted the pediatric neurologist's diagnosis of a rare, incurable genetic disease that was fatal. They consulted a close friend who was a medical researcher, desperately looking for anything to save their toddler's life. The friend told them to gather Lennon's records, saying he would review them and find the best specialist working with mucopolysaccharide diseases.

Greg picked up the medical records from the pediatrician's office, and when Melinda began reviewing them, she realized that Lennon's blood had been abnormal for over a year and that he was severely macrocytic. She immediately called the pediatric neurologist, stating that she thought Lennon had a B_{12} deficiency and asked that he be tested immediately.

Indeed, Melinda was correct—Lennon did have a severe vitamin B_{12} deficiency. Yet none of his doctors suspected or checked him for B_{12} deficiency, despite clear documentation in the medical records that he had exhibited consistently abnormal blood counts, and that he was being breastfed by a lacto-ovo vegetarian mother, which placed him at higher risk for this life-threatening problem.

Lennon's subjective and physical exams shouted out B_{12} deficiency, but all of his doctors missed an easy diagnosis. His serum B_{12} was 130 pg/mL (normal: 211–911), his urinary MMA was 28.9 µmol/L (normal: < 2.4), and his homocysteine was 89.2 µmol/L (normal: 5–15). An even more disturbing fact emerged as Melinda reviewed Lennon's medical records—

she discovered he'd had macrocytic anemia for the past eight months. Lennon also displayed numerous textbook signs and symptoms of pediatric B$_{12}$ deficiency, including developmental delay (motor, speech, language, and social), hypotonia, poor gait, poor growth, poor feeding, failure to thrive, irritability, pallor, anemia, macrocytosis, elevated red cell distribution width, and frequent infections.

As we mentioned in Chapter 8, Melinda remembers bringing up B$_{12}$ deficiency to her pediatrician on three separate occasions. Her pediatrician repeatedly dismissed her input and reassured her that "Nobody gets a B$_{12}$ deficiency. He is getting enough from your milk." When Lennon was 21 months old, the pediatrician stated that his mean corpuscular volume was elevated because he had a metabolic disease—not because of B$_{12}$ deficiency.[1]

Melinda fully trusted her pediatrician, who was the Chief of Pediatrics with a "special interest in nutrition and developmental pediatrics." How could he and all of the other medical and health-care professionals the family encountered fail to make this straightforward diagnosis? But they did.

Lennon finally received B$_{12}$ therapy at the late age of 26 months. He had been symptomatic for over a year, and his brain was actually starving from B$_{12}$ deficiency. His brain MRI (at 22 months of age) revealed atrophy or shrinkage, another telltale sign of B$_{12}$ deficiency. Now 14 years of age, Lennon has speech, language, and cognitive delays. He also has difficulty with fine motor skills. To a casual observer, and even to trained professionals, Lennon's behavior resembles autism. But Lennon does not have autism. He has an acquired brain injury due to B$_{12}$ deficiency—or what would be more accurately labeled as BABI.

Clearly, Lennon was injured by his doctors' repeated failures to diagnose his B$_{12}$ deficiency. But afterward, he was victimized

---

1 Vitamin B$_{12}$ deficiency is actually a metabolic disorder, involved in the metabolism of methylmalonic acid and homocysteine (see Chapter 2). Lennon's pediatrician was sorely uneducated.

a second time by the judicial system. Hired by the Groovers in 2006, Lennon's initial attorney was afraid he could not win the case because he believed the defense would blame Lennon's condition on autism. He told the Groovers, "Autism is the elephant in the room." He said it would be hard for him to prove that the child's brain injury did not stem from autism, and that the defense would use this argument to put doubt in the jurors' minds. When Melinda asked if he would be educating the jurors about B_{12} deficiency, he said that wasn't a good idea because "the jurors' eyes would just glaze over." Judging from his remarks, this attorney himself was completely ignorant about B_{12} deficiency and may have thought that Lennon had autism. His prejudice and failure to understand pediatric B_{12} deficiency ultimately led to his inability to handle the case properly.

The attorney suddenly dropped the case right before trial, forcing the Groovers to find a new attorney, and leaving them only two months to get the next attorney up to speed, find experts to testify, and proceed with the case. The second attorney ultimately lost the case. Unwilling to give up their battle for Lennon and for other children and adults injured by misdiagnosed B_{12} deficiency, the Groovers still had faith in the Alabama justice system and paid an additional $15,000 to appeal their case, taking it to an appellate attorney. Their appeal would reinstate their case and have it proceed to trial.

Eventually, in 2009, the case reached the Supreme Court of Alabama, where two justices ruled in favor of the Groovers. One was opposed, blaming his mother for being a lacto-ovo vegetarian—which was a perfectly healthy choice, had her doctors monitored her B_{12} status and Lennon's and instructed her to supplement her diet with high-dose B_{12} during pregnancy and breastfeeding. And five judges had *no opinion*. The result: no justice for the Groovers, who are now in their 50s and working diligently to find ways to protect their son's future. The Chief Justice of the Supreme Court of Alabama, Sue Bell Cobb, voted in favor of the Groovers, stating that she had "never disagreed more with the Supreme Court."

What does this have to do with making B$_{12}$ deficiency a Never Event? Classifying B$_{12}$ deficiency in this way would make it clear that doctors who fail to check patients like Lennon are negligent. As a result, doctors would begin routinely screening for low B$_{12}$. And if doctors failed in their responsibility, injuring their patients as a result, families would have the entire medical community in their corner when they sought justice.

This was a missed opportunity and a sad day for children all over the world. How could *five* Supreme Court justices have *no opinion*? The Groovers' case could have put B$_{12}$ deficiency in the spotlight, raising awareness and educating health-care professionals and the public about its devastating and injurious consequences. It is too late to prevent Lennon's injury. But it is not too late to help future generations of children and adults by saying "never" to B$_{12}$ deficiency.

WHAT CAN WE DO TO STOP THIS EPIDEMIC IN ITS TRACKS?

- Raise awareness among medical professionals and consumers.
- Identify victims early.
- Test symptomatic and at-risk patients.
- Screen all children with developmental delay or symptoms of autism.
- Screen women during pregnancy and breastfeeding.
- Screen infants at 6 months and 12 months of age using the urinary MMA test.
- Screen all patients diagnosed with depression or other mental illnesses.
- When N$_2$O is used, prescribe high-dose B$_{12}$ before and after administration, after first testing the patient for B$_{12}$ deficiency.

- Educate doctors and dentists to *not* use N_2O in patients with *MTHFR* or *MTRR* mutations.
- Screen all adults age 50 and older.
- Include B_{12} screening in fall-prevention programs.
- Screen all people entering assisted living residences and nursing homes.
- Develop state-of-the-art protocols for identifying and treating B_{12} deficiency.
- Raise the current lower limit of normal serum B_{12} from 200 pg/mL to 500 pg/mL.
- Raise the current daily recommended intake (DRI) of B_{12} for infants, children, and adults, and during pregnancy and breast-feeding.
- Use hydroxo-B_{12} or the active coenzyme forms (methyl-B_{12} and adenosyl-B_{12}) rather than cyano-B_{12} in tablets and lozenges.
- Use hydroxocobalamin injections rather than cyanocobalamin injections, and increase maintenance therapy to bimonthly or trimonthly.
- Pass legislation that recognizes an annual B_{12} Awareness Month.
- Establish B_{12} deficiency as a Never Event.
- Enlist help from government and health-care organizations.
- Enlist help from the media and big businesses.
- Initiate a multimedia campaign—including television ads and public service announcements—designed to raise B_{12} awareness.
- Educate malpractice attorneys.
- Work with other countries to create a Worldwide B_{12} Awareness Day.

What can you do to help combat the epidemic?

Whether you are a parent or a medical professional, we hope you will join us in this battle to save lives, save health-care dollars, and prevent untold numbers of tragedies. Together, we can stop this epidemic in its tracks. This is one of the most preventable and most treatable of all medical scourges—but only if we choose to act.

How can you contribute? Post information about B$_{12}$ deficiency, BABI, and the Autism-B$_{12}$ Connection (ABC) on your Facebook and Twitter accounts. Use mommy groups and women's groups to put the word out on social media. If anyone in your family has suffered as a result of B$_{12}$ deficiency, tell your story publicly.

We cannot simply wait for health-care gatekeepers to put this issue on the table. B$_{12}$ deficiency is health care's dirtiest secret, silently victimizing millions of vulnerable people around the world—particularly children and the elderly. We must bring this secret out into the open by any means possible, from tweets to blogs to Facebook "likes."

When the health-care community fails to protect us, our only choice is to become proactive and protect ourselves and others. So join us in starting a conversation about B$_{12}$ deficiency that will spread around the world, from the streets of New York City, to Toronto, to London, to Rio de Janeiro, to Delhi, to Beijing, to Mexico City, to Cape Town, to Kiev, to Sydney. When millions of us speak up, we will be heard—and we will bring this silent epidemic to an end.

Where can you learn more?

Read our book, *Could It Be B$_{12}$? An Epidemic of Misdiagnoses (2nd edition)*, a comprehensive review of vitamin B$_{12}$ deficiency in persons of all ages.

Online Resources:

- B_{12} Awareness—understanding vitamin B_{12} deficiency (the authors' website): **www.B12Awareness.org**

- **www.B12deficiency.info**

- Pernicious Anaemia/B_{12} Deficiency—support group on Facebook: **www.facebook.com/groups/PAB12DSupportGroup**

- Norman Clinical Laboratory: **www.B12.com**

- View the documentary *Diagnosing and Treating Vitamin B_{12} Deficiency*: **www.youtube.com/watch?feature=player_embedded&v=BvEizypoyO0**

- Check out the feature film *Sally Pacholok*, starring Annet Mahendru. Written, produced, and directed by Elissa Leonard: **www.facebook.com/sallypacholokthemovie**

  Rent or purchase via **vimeo.com** or **amazon.com**

  https://vimeo.com/ondemand/sallypacholokmovie

NURSES SPEAK OUT

Nurses are a vital component of the health-care team. Nurses must become educated about B_{12} deficiency and help facilitate a change in the standard of care. Don't allow your voice to be dismissed. A team effort can change public health-care policy and save lives. Start screening your patients for B_{12} deficiency by using the *Cobalamin Deficiency Risk (CDR) Score* for adults and the *Pediatric Cobalamin Deficiency Risk (PCDR) Score* for children (see Appendices A and B). If your patient is at risk or symptomatic, be that person's advocate and notify his or her doctor as well as your clinical manager. Begin documenting the incidence of low B_{12} and B_{12} deficiency at your facility. When nurses are involved in decision-making policies, patient outcomes improve, the community benefits, and costs decrease.

Appendices

APPENDIX A: COBALAMIN DEFICIENCY RISK (CDR) SCORE

COBALAMIN DEFICIENCY RISK (CDR SCORE)

Low risk:	0–1
At risk:	2–4
High risk:	5 or greater

I. NEUROLOGICAL MANIFESTATIONS (+2 EACH)
- Paresthesias
- Weakness of legs, arms, or trunk
- Unsteady gait, balance problems
- Ataxia
- Dizziness or lightheadedness
- Tremors
- Restless legs
- Lhermitte's sign
- Romberg's sign
- Abnormal Babinski reflex
- Visual disturbances
- Forgetfulness, short-term memory loss, or dementia
- Mental status changes
- Impotence, erectile dysfunction
- Urinary or fecal incontinence
- Impaired vibration, position sense
- Abnormal reflexes
- Seizures
- Paralysis

II. NEUROPSYCHIATRIC MANIFESTATIONS (+2 EACH)
- Depression, suicidal ideations
- Diagnosis of mental illness or on psychiatric medications
- Postpartum depression or psychosis
- Anxiety
- Poor concentration or foggy thinking
- ADD/ADHD
- Personality changes
- Irritability
- Paranoia
- Mania
- Hallucinations
- Psychosis
- Violent behavior
- Homicidal ideations

III. HEMATOLOGIC MANIFESTATIONS (+2 EACH)
- Anemia
- Macrocytosis
- Hypersegmented neutrophils
- Anisocytosis
- Leukopenia
- Thrombocytopenia
- Pancytopenia

IV. GENERAL SIGNS/SYMPTOMS (+1 EACH)
- Generalized weakness or fatigue
- Shortness of breath
- Pallor or jaundice
- Frequent falls or near falls
- Loss of appetite/weight loss
- Frequent infections, poor wound healing
- Orthostatic hypotension
- Postural orthostatic tachycardia
- Occlusive vascular disorder or thrombotic events (e.g., PE, DVT, CVA, MI, portal vein thrombosis)
- Cervical dysplasia
- Intrauterine growth retardation
- Malnutrition
- Glossitis
- Tinnitus
- Skin hyperpigmentation or hypopigmentation
- Hepatomegaly or splenomegaly

V. GASTROINTESTINAL RISKS (+2 EACH)
- Decreased stomach acid or atrophic gastritis
- Gastroparesis
- *Helicobacter pylori* infection
- Giardiasis
- GERD or ulcer disease
- Gastrectomy (partial or complete), bariatric surgery
- Ileal resection (partial or complete)
- Malabsorption syndromes (e.g., Crohn's disease, IBS, celiac disease)
- Pancreatitis, pancreatic exocrine insufficiency
- Small intestinal bacterial overgrowth
- *Diphyllobothrium latum* (fish tapeworm)
- Liver disease

VI. (a) POPULATION AT RISK (+2 EACH)
- Vegans, vegetarians, macrobiotic diets
- MTHFR gene mutation
- Nitrous oxide administration or abuse
- Eating disorders

(b) POPULATION AT RISK (+1 EACH)
- Age 50 or over
- Pregnancy
- Intrauterine growth retardation
- Autoimmune disorders (e.g., thyroid, IDDM, lupus)
- Family history of pernicious anemia
- Proton-pump inhibitor or H2-blocker use
- Metformin use
- Alcoholism
- Dialysis patients
- AIDS
- Chemo- or radiation therapy
- Phenylketonuria (PKU)
- Down syndrome

Appendix B: Pediatric Cobalamin Deficiency Risk (PCDR) Score

Pediatric Cobalamin Deficiency Risk (PCDR Score)

Low risk: 0–1
At risk: 2–4
High risk: 5 or greater

I. Neurological Manifestations (+2 each)
- Developmental delay or regression (motor, speech, language, or social)
- Hypotonia
- Poor suckling/swallowing
- Abnormal movements
- Ataxia
- Tremors
- Seizures
- Paresthesias
- Lhermitte's sign
- Romberg's sign
- Weakness of extremities
- Clumsiness or falling
- Dizziness
- Visual disturbances
- Impaired vibration, position sense
- Mental status changes
- Abnormal reflexes
- Paralysis
- Coma

II. Neuropsychiatric Manifestations (+2 each)
- Depression or apathy
- Suicidal ideations
- Diagnosis of mental illness or on psychiatric medications
- Anxiety
- ADD/ADHD
- Personality changes
- Poor concentration, foggy thinking
- Poor verbal fluency or problem solving
- Low IQ
- Paranoia
- Mania
- Hallucinations
- Psychosis
- Violent behavior or homicidal ideations

III. Hematologic Manifestations (+2 each)
- Anemia
- Macrocytosis
- Hypersegmented neutrophils
- Anisocytosis
- Leukopenia
- Thrombocytopenia
- Pancytopenia

IV. General Signs/Symptoms (+1 each)
- Abnormal head circumference or growth
- Anorexia, poor feeding/appetite
- Drowsiness or lethargy
- Dyspnea
- Failure to thrive

- Frequent infections
- Glossitis or stomatitis
- Hepatomegaly or splenomegaly
- Irritability
- Orthostatic hypotension
- Pallor or jaundice
- Postural orthostatic tachycardia syndrome (POTS)
- Skin hyperpigmentation or hypopigmentation
- Systolic flow murmur
- Tinnitus
- Chronic vomiting or diarrhea
- Weakness or fatigue
- Weight loss or weight <25th percentile

V. Gastrointestinal Risks (+2 each)
- Malabsorption syndromes (e.g., Crohn's disease, IBS, celiac disease, gluten sensitivity)
- GERD
- Gastroparesis
- *Helicobacter pylori* infection
- Giardiasis
- Gastrectomy (partial or complete)
- Ileal resection (partial or complete)
- Small intestinal bacterial overgrowth
- Pancreatitis, pancreatic exocrine insufficiency
- Liver disease
- *Diphyllobothrium latum* (fish tapeworm)

VI. (a) Population at Risk (+2 each)
- Vegans, vegetarians, macrobiotic diets (mother or child)
- MTHFR gene mutation
- Nitrous oxide administration or abuse
- Eating disorders

(b) Population at Risk (+1 each)
- Proton-pump inhibitor or H2-blocker use
- Metformin use
- Breastfed children
- Pregnancy (teens)
- Family history of pernicious anemia
- Autoimmune disorders
- AIDS
- Chemo- or radiation therapy
- Low birth weight
- NTD, cleft lip/palate, or congenital heart defect
- Hydrocephalus
- Phenylketonuria (PKU)
- Down syndrome

Appendix C: Signs and Symptoms of Inborn Errors of B12 Metabolism*

I. Neurological Manifestations
- Hypotonia
- Abnormal or absent reflexes
- Poor suckling or swallowing
- Infantile spasms
- Tremors
- Seizures
- Global developmental delay
- Encephalopathy
- Retinopathy
- Nystagmus
- Coma

II. Hematologic Manifestations
- Anemia
- Macrocytosis
- Hypersegmented neutrophils
- Anisocytosis
- Leukopenia
- Thrombocytopenia
- Pancytopenia

III. General Signs/Symptoms
- Poor head growth
- Microcephaly
- Hydrocephalus
- Low birth weight
- Intrauterine growth retardation
- Poor feeding
- Atrophic stomatitis
- Glossitis
- Anorexia
- Vomiting
- Failure to thrive
- Drowsiness or lethargy
- Dyspnea
- Glossitis
- Hepatomegaly
- Splenomegaly
- Irritability
- Pallor or jaundice
- Systolic flow murmur

IV. Metabolic
- Metabolic acidosis
- Ketonuria
- Hyperammonemia

V. Congenital Defects— Associated Conditions
- Congenital heart defect
- Neural tube defect
- Cleft lip or palate
- Hemolytic uremic syndrome**

*The signs and symptoms can also be seen in infants and children with severe vitamin B_{12} deficiency without an inborn error in B_{12} metabolism.

** Can be easily confused with Cobalamin-C. Ask if this disorder occurs in any siblings. If so, all siblings need testing.

187

Appendix D: Causes of B12 Deficiency

I. General
- Decreased stomach acid
- Atrophic gastritis
- Autoimmune pernicious anemia
- *Helicobacter pylori*
- Gastrectomy (partial or complete)
- Gastric bypass surgery (weight loss)
- Ileal resection (partial or complete)
- Gastrointestinal neoplasms
- Malnutrition
- Inadequate diet
- Vegan, vegetarian, lacto-ovo vegetarian, macrobiotic diets (without proper supplementation)
- Eating disorders
- Poor diet (junk food, processed foods)
- Atypical diets (phenylketonuria diet)
- Malabsorption syndromes
- Celiac disease (gluten enteropathy)
- Crohn's disease
- *Diphyllobothrium* infection
- Giardiasis
- Blind loop syndrome
- Inflammatory bowel disease
- Small bowel overgrowth
- Alcoholism
- Radiation therapy
- Inborn errors of B$_{12}$ metabolism
- Transcobalamin II deficiency
- Pancreatic exocrine insufficiency
- Imerslund-Gräesbeck syndrome
- Zollinger-Ellison syndrome
- Liver disease

II. Drug Induced
- Antacids
- Chemotherapy
- Cholestyramine (Questran)
- Colchicine
- H2- blockers (Zantac, Tagamet, Pepcid)
- Metformin (Glucophage)
- Mycifradin sulfate (Neomycin)
- Nitrous oxide (anesthesia or abuse)
- Para-aminosalicylates
- Phenytoin (Dilantin)
- Potassium chloride (K-Dur)
- Proton-pump inhibitors (Prilosec, Nexium, Prevacid, Protonix)
- Valproic acid (Depakote)

III. Increased Demands
- Breastfeeding
- Chronic hemolytic anemia
- Hyperthyroidism
- Multiple myeloma
- Myeloproliferative disorders
- Neoplasms
- Pregnancy

APPENDIX E: WHOM TO TEST AND WHO IS AT RISK FOR B12 DEFICIENCY

- Developmental delay in infants or children
- Developmental regression in infants or children
- Diagnosis of cerebral palsy
- Neurological or motor symptoms
- Mental status changes
- Depression
- Suicidal or homicidal ideations
- Diagnosis of mental illness
- Diagnosis of learning disabilities
- Diagnosis of autism spectrum disorders
- Pregnant and nursing mothers
- Breastfed infants of symptomatic or at-risk mothers
- MTHFR gene mutation
- Diagnosis of any type of dementia
- Gastrointestinal disorders
- Gastrointestinal surgeries
- Gastric bypass patients
- Anemia
- Macrocytosis
- Iron deficiency anemia
- Sickle cell anemia
- Postural orthostatic tachycardia syndrome (POTS)
- Vegans, vegetarians, macrobiotic diets
- Age 50 and over
- Autoimmune disorders
- Family history of pernicious anemia
- Proton-pump inhibitor use
- Metformin use
- Anticonvulsant use
- Diabetics
- Cancer patients—chemotherapy and radiation therapy
- Visual disturbances (optic neuritis, atrophy, macular degeneration)

APPENDIX F: DISORDERS WITH POSSIBLE UNDERLYING OR MISDIAGNOSED B12 DEFICIENCY

- Autism spectrum disorders
- Pervasive developmental disorders
- Cerebral palsy
- Depression
- Postpartum depression/psychosis
- Any psychiatric disorder
- Dementia
- Alzheimer's disease
- Frontotemporal dementia
- Vertigo
- Anemia
- Multiple sclerosis
- Amyotrophic lateral sclerosis (ALS)
- Guillain-Barré syndrome
- Parkinson's disease
- Essential tremor
- Peripheral neuropathies (e.g., diabetic, CIDP)
- Other neurological disorders
- Restless leg syndrome
- Postural orthostatic tachycardia syndrome (POTS)
- Radiculopathy
- Chronic pain disorder
- Chronic fatigue syndrome
- Fibromyalgia
- Erectile dysfunction
- Infertility
- Congestive heart failure
- AIDS dementia complex
- Occlusive vascular disorders or thrombotic events

APPENDIX G: SIGNS AND SYMPTOMS OF B12 DEFICIENCY BLAMED ON AUTISM SPECTRUM DISORDER

- Developmental delay
- Developmental regression
- Speech or language delay
- Communication problems
- Social delay
- Reduced IQ
- Intellectual disability
- Abnormal fine and gross motor movement
- Flapping
- Fixation with spinning objects
- Stimming
- Aloof or withdrawn behavior
- Seizures
- Visual disturbances
- Poor immune response to vaccinations

APPENDIX H: LABORATORY AND OTHER TESTS TO AID IN THE DIAGNOSIS OF B12 DEFICIENCY

- Serum B$_{12}$
- Urine or serum methylmalonic acid (MMA)
- Homocysteine
- Holotranscobalamin II (HoloTC)
- Gastrin
- Parietal cell antibody
- Intrinsic factor antibody
- Gastric secretion analysis (pH)
- Peripheral blood smear
- MTHFR-2 gene mutation
- MRI or CT of the brain
- MRI spine
- Evoked potentials
- Electroencephalography (EEG)
- Tilt table test

APPENDIX I: WHY B12 DEFICIENCY IS AN EPIDEMIC

- Knowledge deficit among physicians and other health-care providers
- Poor or absent screening in symptomatic and at-risk patients
- Clinicians ignoring the neurological and psychiatric manifestations of B12 deficiency
- Current range for "normal" serum B12 set far too low
- Clinicians not using other adjunctive diagnostic B12 tests (e.g., urinary methylmalonic acid)
- Clinicians not treating symptomatic patients whose serum B12 levels fall in the gray zone (200–500 pg/mL)
- Clinicians waiting for enlarged red blood cells or macrocytic anemia to be present before testing or treating patients
- B12 screening not provided for symptomatic children with developmental delay/regression or with a diagnosis on the autism spectrum
- Women and children not being screened for *MTHFR* gene mutation
- B12 screening not performed during preconception or pregnancy, or during breastfeeding
- B12 screening not provided for patients presenting with mental illness or in medical clearance prior to psychiatric evaluation
- B12 screening not provided for older adults who fall or are at risk for falling
- B12 screening not provided for older adults with cognitive changes or dementia

APPENDIX J: NEUROPSYCHIATRIC MANIFESTATIONS OF PEDIATRIC B12 DEFICIENCY

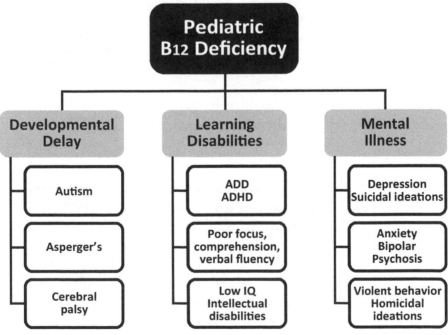

191

APPENDIX K: CAUSES OF B12 DEFICIENCY IN CHILDREN

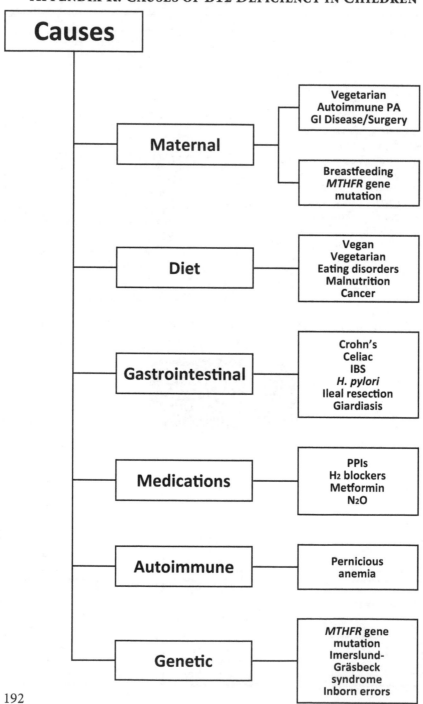

APPENDIX L: CHILD AT HIGH RISK FOR B12 DEFICIENCY

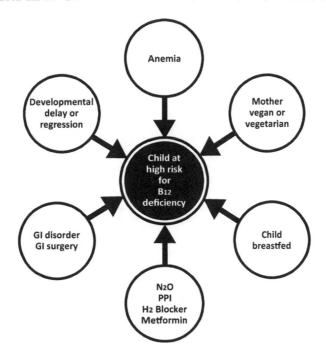

APPENDIX M: THIS INFANT/TODDLER NEEDS B12 TESTING

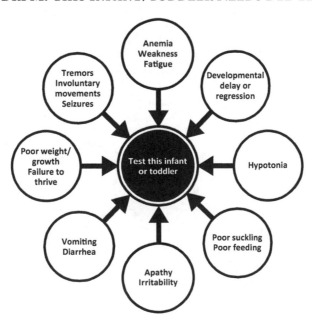

Appendix N: This Child or Teen Needs B12 Testing

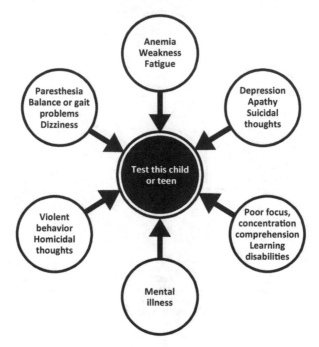

Appendix O: This Child Is at Risk for Misdiagnosed B12 Deficiency

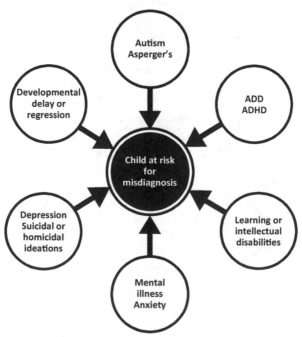

APPENDIX P: HIGH-RISK WOMAN DURING PRECONCEPTION, PREGNANCY, OR BREASTFEEDING: EACH VARIABLE LISTED BELOW INCREASES MOM'S RISK FOR B12 DEFICIENCY AND BABI IN HER CHILD.

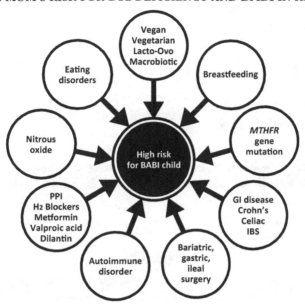

APPENDIX Q: NEUROPATHOPHYSIOLOGY OF VITAMIN B12 DEFICIENCY.

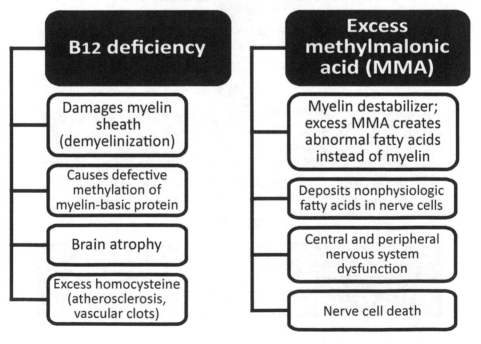

APPENDIX R: WHEN B12 DEFICIENCY CAUSES SCD:
SUBACUTE (SYMPTOMS DEVELOP SLOWLY)
COMBINED (MULTIPLE NEUROLOGIC SYSTEMS AFFECTED)
DEGENERATION (NERVE CELLS ARE BEING DESTROYED).

Subacute combined degeneration

Central Nervous System (brain, spinal cord)	Peripheral Nervous System	Autonomic Nervous System

Myelin sheath damaged or destroyed

Degeneration of axons (nerves)	Cognitive disturbances Brain atrophy Dementia

Posterior and lateral column disease

↓ Fine touch	Sympathetic nervous system dysfunction ↓ Proprioception

Spinothalamic tract disease

↓ Touch	↓ Pain	↓ Temperature	↓ Sensation

Disturbed neurotransmitters
Peripheral neuropathy
Myeloneuropathy

Depression Psychosis	Incontinence Impotence	Nerve death Paralysis

Paresthesias, clumsy movement, ataxia, limb weakness, visual problems, unsteady gait, balance disorders, spasticity, confusion, mental illness

Index

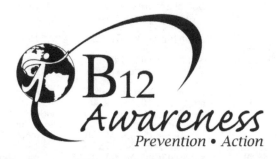

MISSION STATEMENT: UNMASKING THE EPIDEMIC OF UNDIAGNOSED VITAMIN B_{12} DEFICIENCY THROUGH EDUCATION, PREVENTION, AND ADVOCACY.

B_{12} AWARENESS GOALS:

1. Raise awareness of the dangers of B_{12} deficiency by reeducating the medical community and educating the public.

2. Promote early diagnosis and treatment to prevent neurological and cognitive injury, disability, poor outcomes, and premature death.

3. Educate society and health-care professionals on the role B_{12} deficiency plays in poor overall health, developmental and intellectual disabilities, cognitive decline, dementia, fall-related trauma, neurologic injury, mental illness, anemia, and vascular occlusions.

4. Promote screening during pregnancy and breastfeeding.

5. Promote screening of infants and children.

6. Promote screening of older adults and psychiatric patients.

7. Enlist help from the public, the media, Congress, governmental agencies, health-care organizations, and attorneys to expose and eliminate billions of dollars of waste in the health-care system due to undiagnosed B_{12} deficiency.

8. Promote health, protect the public, and save lives.

9. Promote further research.

10. Pass legislation in the U.S. that recognizes September as B_{12} Awareness Month.

11. Work with other countries to create a Worldwide B_{12} Awareness Day.

WWW.B12AWARENESS.ORG

OTHER INFORMATIVE B_{12} WEBSITES:
- www.b12deficiency.info (U.K.)
- www.B12.com (U.S.)

About the Authors

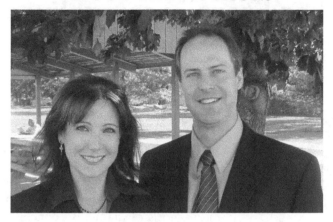

Sally Pacholok has 37 years of experience in the health-care field. For the past 29 years, she has practiced emergency nursing in addition to conducting extensive research into B_{12} deficiency. She is a frequent guest on nationally syndicated talk shows, a lecturer, and the co-author of *Could It Be B_{12}? An Epidemic of Misdiagnoses* (2nd edition, 2011)—the winner of the Indie Excellence Award for best health book. *Could It Be B_{12}?* has been translated into Bulgarian, Dutch, German, Italian, Slovenian, and Spanish.

Pacholok educates the public and health-care professionals worldwide about B_{12} deficiency, and has appeared in two documentaries. In 2014, film producer Elissa Leonard wrote and directed the movie *Sally Pacholok*, which is based on Pacholok's life-long battle to raise awareness about B_{12} deficiency and the consequences of its misdiagnosis. In 2009, Sally and Dr. Jeffrey Stuart created B_{12} Awareness (**www.B12Awareness.org**).

Pacholok received her bachelor's degree in nursing from Wayne State University in Detroit, Michigan. She is an Advanced Cardiac Life Support (ACLS) provider and has assisted instructors at a local college in training paramedics in ACLS. She is a Trauma Nursing Core Course (TNCC) provider, an Emergency Nurse Pediatric Course (ENPC) provider, and a member of the Emergency Nurses Association (ENA).

Jeffrey J. Stuart, D.O., is a board-certified emergency medicine physician with 23 years' experience in the specialty. He is also certified in Advanced Trauma Life Support (ATLS), Advanced Cardiac Life Support (ACLS), and Pediatric Advanced Life Support (PALS). Stuart received his Doctor of Osteopathy degree from the Chicago College of Osteopathic Medicine in Downers Grove, Illinois. He is a member of the American Osteopathic Association, the American College of Osteopathic Emergency Physicians, the Michigan Osteopathic Association, and the Macomb County Osteopathic Medical Association.

Sally and Jeff were married in 1994 and reside in Shelby Township, Michigan.

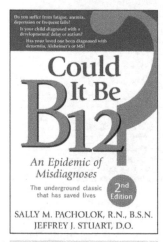
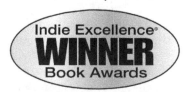

Now an award-winning film starring Annet Mahendru as Sally Pacholok

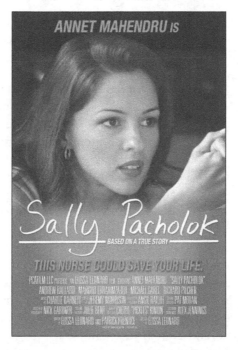

See the amazing true story behind the book *Could It Be B12?* Starring Annet Mahendru (*The Americans*) as Sally Pacholok, **Sally Pacholok** tells the real-life story of how an emergency room nurse uncovered a health threat to her patients … and then grew determined to educate the world about the dangers of B12 deficiency. An inspiring story about how one woman has saved lives by speaking truth to power, **Sally Pacholok** shows how a single individual can make a big difference — and it will make you want to stand up and cheer!

Winner Best Feature DC Independent Film Festival

Winner of Ten Television Internet and Video Association Peer Awards

See the movie at Vimeo.com or buy today at Amazon.com

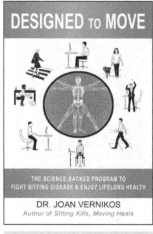

Printed in the USA
CPSIA information can be obtained
at www.ICGtesting.com
JSHW082202140824
68134JS00014B/371

9 781610 352871